Busted!

THE
Fab FOUNDATIONS™
GUIDE TO BRAS THAT
FIT, FLATTER AND FEEL FANTASTIC

ALI CUDBY
America's #1 Bra Coach

Busted!

Advance Praise

"Busted examines why the fit of a woman's bra is not only incredibly complicated, but also integral to good health. Author Ali Cudby finally solves the bra fit conundrum with easy humor and deep knowledge, then explains how to address those issues successfully."

—JEFFREY KLUGER, NEW YORK TIMES BESTSELLING AUTHOR OF APOLLO 13 AND THE SIBLING EFFECT

"A bra is one of the most misunderstood parts of a woman's wardrobe. Fortunately, Ali is here to change all that! Her debut book not only lifts bust lines; it also lifts spirits, with a reassuring yet informative style that's perfect for all your bra questions."

—TREACLE, THE LINGERIE ADDICT, WORLD'S #1 LINGERIE BLOG

"Can a bra change a life? The answer is yes, and Ali Cudby has crafted a wonderful book that will resonate with women looking to change not only their wardrobe but their lives. Busted! is truly uplifting—full of solid advice and personal stories that readers will find illuminating, insightful, and hard to put down."

—LUIS PAREDES, PUBLISHER AND FOUNDER OF THELINGERIEJOURNAL.COM, AN ONLINE RESOURCE AND PUBLICATION FOR THE LINGERIE INDUSTRY

Advance Praise

"Ali's book makes you want to go bra shopping, just so you can use her amazing advice to finally find that perfect bra!"

—ELLEN SHING, LULA LU PETITE LINGERIE

"If you want a PICTURE PERFECT fit with comfort and style, Busted! is a must-read. Picture this: Ali Cudby has taken a difficult topic and made it simple."

—HOWARD SHAPIRO M.D., NEW YORK TIMES BESTSELLING AUTHOR OF THE PICTURE PERFECT WEIGHT LOSS SERIES

"Ali Cudby is a one-of-a-kind genius and a gift to every woman (and man!) alive. If you want to look thinner, eliminate neck or back pain and wear your clothes with confidence, then you need Ali. If you've got dozens of bras that are sitting in your drawer collecting dust, then you need Ali. If you care about your breast health, then you need Ali. Seriously – don't buy one more bra until you read Busted!"

—WENDY LIPTON-DIBNER, BESTSELLING AUTHOR OF SHATTER YOUR SPEED LIMITS™: FAST-TRACK YOUR SUCCESS AND GET WHAT YOU TRULY WANT IN BUSINESS AND IN LIFE AND FOUNDER OF THE MOVE PEOPLE TO ACTION SYSTEM FOR EXPERTS, AUTHORS AND ENTREPRENEURS™

Busted!

THE
$\mathcal{F}ab$ FOUNDATIONS™
GUIDE TO BRAS THAT
FIT, FLATTER AND FEEL FANTASTIC

ALI CUDBY
America's #1 Bra Coach

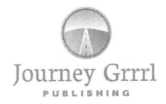

Journey Grrrl
PUBLISHING

Published in the United States by Journey Grrrl Publishing

ISBN: 978-1-9369-8404-6
Library of Congress Control Number: 2011934597

Interior Design by Karen Leigh Burton/Poodles Doodles
Cover Design by Abby Weintraub
Cover art: Imagezoo/Getty Images
Fab Girl Illustrations by Judith Shakes Design
Headshot of Ali Cudby courtesy of Brian K. Donnelly

To Joe,

My Aphrodisiac Is You

Table of Contents

My mission is to help every woman understand how a bra should fit her unique body, so she can enjoy a lifetime of Fab Foundations™.

— Ali Cudby

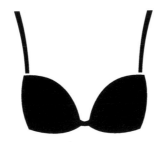

Introduction
Tears in the Fitting Room

I was a late bloomer. As a young teen in summer camp, I was teased for being flat-chested. Eventually, I started developing in eighth grade, and once I started growing, I didn't stop. During my high school years, I went from average to busty to huge. I joked to my friends that I had a six-pack: two resting in my bra, two spilling over the top, and two sliding beneath the underwire.

Bra shopping felt like an act of masochism. The largest bra I could find at our local department store was a DD, and it didn't come close to fitting. I'm sure the saleslady felt sorry for me. When I did find a bra that sort of worked, it was always something resembling a flak jacket. As a teenager, all I wanted was lacy lingerie in pretty colors, but there was nothing available in my size.

Every time I went shopping, I couldn't help hoping that the stores would have something new. I was always disappointed, and no matter how much I steeled myself beforehand, I always ended up crying in the fitting room.

These shopping experiences made me feel humiliated, as if each bra that didn't fit was communicating a larger message: that I didn't fit. Although I excelled in lots of areas, failing to feel good about my body compromised my self-esteem and undermined my confidence on the dating scene.

After years of insecurity and adolescent heartache, I had breast reduction surgery during my freshman year of college. Although they removed half of my breast mass I was still a D cup. I could finally walk into just about any lingerie department and find a bra my size! While bra shopping was great, the surgery did not restore my self-esteem as effectively as I had hoped. I was satisfied with my bra selection, but I was still unhappy with my body.

Inevitably, I gained weight, and the extra pounds found their way to my chest. It didn't take long before I was right back where I had been throughout high school: not fitting into any of the bras available in an average department store. Once again, I found myself crying in the fitting room. As I transitioned through my twenties, I figured out other ways to feel good about myself. I focused on my career and friends and eventually came to embrace my curves.

I began dating a charming Englishman who, before long, insisted it was time to meet his family on the other side of the pond. On a whirlwind weekend in England, we were walking through lovely, historic Cambridge with my boyfriend's family when I spied the marquee of my dreams.

Bravissimo—For Big-Boobed Girls was a shop made in heaven. It was like a beacon of light entering my body, drawing me in. As I veered in closer to look at the merchandise, I couldn't help myself. Without thinking, I went inside, leaving my boyfriend's family standing on the sidewalk, wondering what had come over me.

As I entered the store, I had to wonder, too. I consider myself a strong, independent woman. I've owned my own businesses and have done amazing things in my life (including marrying that charming Englishman). It may seem overblown to say that finding a store with properly fitted bras was life changing, but it was.

Up until that day, I had always felt uncomfortable— physically and emotionally—adjusting my bra all day long while waiting desperately for the moment I could rip it off at night. Over the years, dents had formed in my shoulders from the tight bra straps holding up my chest, and even worse, I was constantly self-conscious in my skin.

But Bravissimo changed all that. It was filled with bras that were pretty, lacy, feminine—and all in large cup sizes. I received a professional fitting and bought bras in a size I never knew existed. Even better, the lovely fitter brought me a dozen gorgeous bras to try on. With each new garment, I felt more and more whole. All of a sudden, I noticed myself standing straighter. I was actually lifted for the first time in my life in a bra that was also nice to touch and attractive to look at.

I already looked better in my clothes and the bras felt so comfortable! I never realized they could feel so good! I imagined I wouldn't have to think about my bra anymore during the day once I put it on in the morning. More important, with the right bra, I could begin to focus on more important aspects of my life without distraction.

While my future family stood outside, wondering what kind of wacky American girl their boy had brought home, I was experiencing the most remarkable revelation. Once again, just as I had so many times before, I found myself crying in the dressing room — except this time they were tears of joy.

On that day, I knew I would never wear uncomfortable, ill-fitting bras again. I got home and began talking to my friends, only to realize that whether they had grapes or melons, almost none of them had bras that fit. In fact, most of them said, "I know my bra doesn't fit!" When I heard them, I was floored. For all those years, I had suffered in silence, thinking I was the lone oddball. How could so many smart, successful women have ill-fitting bras? Then it struck me — as women, we never really learn how a bra *should* fit.

I resolved to start fitting my friends. The more I helped, the more people asked for a turn. All of a sudden, it was like that old shampoo commercial. Every woman I helped told their two friends — and so on, and so on. But working with my circle of friends wasn't enough. I wanted *every* woman to look and feel amazing, and that was the ultimate inspiration for this book.

As I like to say, a bra is like a house. Without a solid foundation, everything sags. That's why bras are called foundation garments, and it's why I named my company Fab Foundations™.

The fruits of all my labors fitting women and studying the field has been distilled into a series of steps I call The FabFit™ Formula. It is the heart of this book.

Using The FabFit™ Formula, you will acquire skills and valuable information that can last a lifetime, even as your body changes. These include how to fit a bra correctly, find the garment you prefer, and shop strategically, thereby saving money, stress, and time — all key factors in promoting a healthier lifestyle. Because when you wear the wrong size bra day after day, year after year, there are consequences for your health, both physically and emotionally.

Once you've completed this book, you will be able to put on a bra in the morning that fits correctly and enjoy leaving it alone and have it remain comfortable all day until you take it off at night. Imagine standing straighter, looking better in your clothes, and appearing 10 pounds thinner. That's what FabFit™ can do for you.

You will no longer have to endure the discomfort and indignity of bras that don't fit. You, too, can join the club of healthy and happy women who are enjoying a lifetime of Fab Foundations™.

The Fab Fit™ Formula

- *Your best bra fit is an important part of your physical and emotional health.*

- *Bodies are not one-size-fits-all so bra measurement systems shouldn't be either.*

- *Focus on fit instead of size.*

- *Assess your fit in the band, cup, bridge, and straps.*

- *Determine your body type.*

- *Always try on a bra to know how it fits your unique body.*

- *Buy fewer bras of better quality.*

- *Take care of your bras to get the most mileage for your money.*

Every woman needs—no, deserves—a properly fitting bra. Not only does it make a profound difference in the way you look & feel; the simple truth is that your clothes simply won't work their best without one, no matter how much you may have spent on them.

—Treacle, The Lingerie Addict,
World's #1 Lingerie Blog

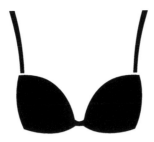

1

Fit's Not Rocket Science: It's Harder!

When it comes to finding the right bra—one that fits correctly, feels comfortable, and can make you look much thinner—it shouldn't be an epic battle. When you read fashion magazines or websites, it seems like finding your bra size is easy. A little more investigation reveals that there are a lot of different methods to fit a bra, and many of them are contradictory. In fact, the entire philosophy of bra sizing is confusing.

Mad Men Determined Our Bra Size

Some of the confusion goes back to World War II, when band and cup sizing became the norm. The perfect hourglass figure was considered to be 36-26-36. The first measurement was supposed to represent the bust size, so women seeking that hourglass ideal wanted to buy a bra that reinforced the idea that they were "a 36."

The problem was that the measurement actually corresponded to the over the bust measurement, not the band size. In reality, that 36-26-36 woman actually had a band size that measured somewhere around 32 inches.

The geniuses on Madison Avenue thought it would be confusing for women to think of themselves as a 32 when so much of the hype was based upon a size 36 being the ideal. So they came up with a methodology that became the norm: to ascertain band size, first you measure your body under the bust, then add four to five inches. So, essentially, women have an incredibly confusing process for measuring bra band size based on a marketing gimmick.

The Three Biggest Myths of Bra Sizing

Let's begin by debunking the three biggest myths concerning bra size.

Myth 1: You don't fit.

That is simply not true. There is a bra out there for virtually everybody, and this book tells you how to find it.

Myth 2: Once you find your bra size, you are done.

In fact, bra size is a moving target. Ask any growing teenager, new mother, or mature woman. Bodies change and bra sizes right along with them.

Myth 3: It's easy to find your bra size.

Simply put—it's not. If you have ever adjusted a slipping bra strap, felt uncomfortable in your bra, or wished for a better silhouette, then you know that the quest for the ideal bra can feel hopeless.

The Search for a Bra Can Feel Like a Bust

Anita, a 38-year-old mother of two, knew she needed to go bra shopping, but she couldn't find anything in local stores that fit her properly. Feeling embarrassed and overwhelmed, she let her ill-fitting DD bras fall into tatters. That made it exceedingly difficult for Anita to feel professional in the clothes she wore each day, working as a bank teller.

Christina, a 24-year-old schoolteacher, had been hearing the same refrain for years from the sales ladies at the mall. Whenever they spotted her petite frame, they told her to shop for training bras in the children's department, or worse, they suggested that she didn't need a bra at all. Christina, a former gymnast, was too small for adult lingerie, which ultimately made her feel less like a woman.

Maggie, a 45-year-old lawyer, looked at her chest one night after a long day of work and childcare and felt utterly deflated, much like her breasts after nursing two babies. Without knowing any better, she continued wearing her 34B bras and assumed the sagging was a reality she would just have to accept.

Recognize anyone you know?

Anita, Christina, and Maggie are typical of the millions of American women who face daily issues with their bras. They may be successful and happy in their day-to-day lives, but when they walk into a lingerie department it's a different story. These women represent a majority who may not like their bra size or breast shape or simply may not know what size to wear. As a result, they certainly don't enjoy shopping for bras or like how they fit. All too often, bra shopping makes these women feel like there's something wrong with them or their bodies.

But finding a bra that fits and makes you feel good can make rocket science seem easy; at least it follows a formula. Confusion about bra size explains why industry studies consistently show that somewhere between 70 and 85 percent of women are wearing the wrong bra size. That amounts to between 80 and 100 million women over the age of 18. And the statistics for younger girls are even worse.

It doesn't have to be this way. Most, if not all, of the reasons these women are still struggling with finding the right bra are due to incomplete and misguided information. And some of the information out there is flat-out wrong.

Finding the Right Bra Is Hard!

Anita's bra straps constantly fell off her shoulders, and she often readjusted them, even during meetings in her office.

When the time came for her performance review, her manager took issue with Anita's "constant fidgeting," as if it compromised her professionalism. Even though it was never specifically mentioned, Anita knew the culprits were her ill-fitting bras. Unable to find anything that fit, Anita felt sloppy, in her life and at work.

Because there are few industry standards for sizing, confusion about how to take a measurement, and inconsistent training of in-store fitters, women continue to be handicapped in their search for the proper fitting bra.

Finding the right bra is not easy! It requires compassionate, professional advice, which you can find right here. So join the club. Like millions of other women, there is nothing wrong with you. You just haven't found the right bra for you — yet.

But you will.

After Anita, Christina, and Maggie had the pleasure of being professionally fitted, their situations improved significantly. Now Anita proudly wears a 42H, and for the first time in her life, has pretty bras that make her feel better rather than worse. Christina found a range of companies that design bras expressly for her petite body type. She no longer feels banished to the girls' department. Maggie found a more supportive bra that gave her the lift to look and feel like her pre-baby days.

So let's get started on the journey to your own FabFit™! The first step is to take a good, hard look at your current bras. Please examine The FabFit™ Personal Assessment to see what's relevant for you.

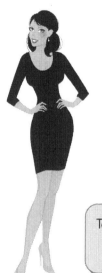

To download a printable copy of your own
FabFit™ Personal Assessment, go to
www.fabfoundations.com/bustedextras

The FabFit™ Personal Assessment

Before determining your bra size, think about how your bra fits. These questions may help you identify what you need to change.

1. Is your bra uncomfortable?
2. Do your bra straps dig into your shoulders?
3. Do your bra straps ever slip off your shoulders?
4. Does your underwire poke into your breasts?
5. Over the course of a day, does your bra band creep up your back?
6. Does your breast tissue spill over the cups of your bra?
7. Does your breast tissue fall out the bottom of your bra cups?
8. Is there any gap between your bra and your body?
9. How about when you raise your arms?
10. Is there any gap between the middle portion of your bra (between your breasts) and your body?
11. Have you gained or lost more than 10 pounds without being re-fitted?
12. Do your bra cups wrinkle or stand away from your body?
13. Do you have back fat and/or bulges at the bra band?
14. Do your breasts appear to sag in your bra?
15. Do you have divots or ridges in your shoulders, where your bra straps sit?
16. Is there a hump in your upper back, between your shoulders?

If you answered YES to any of these questions, then your bra probably does not fit you properly. Keep reading! The next few chapters will help you figure it out.

Wearing a bra is a health thing to keep breast tissue supported. You have children, your body changes. You can't be the same as you were when you were eighteen.

—Emily Lau, Owner, The Little Bra Company

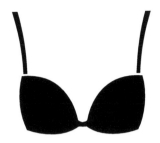

2

WARNING!
The Wrong Bra
Can Be Hazardous to
Your Health

Every day like clockwork, Kate got a headache. It usually started during the late morning, as her workday intensified, when she felt as if her chest were being squeezed—which it was. Why? Her bra was too tight—as always. Kate didn't even realize that her too-small band was the culprit; she just knew that her performance at work was suffering and that she came home every day too drained to play with her three small children. To make matters worse, she went to bed every night feeling exhausted, frustrated, and guilty.

Laura trudged to her chiropractor every Friday to get an adjustment. She was tired of spending the time and money at the doctor each week, but her chronic back pain left her no other option. Her large breasts were heavy, and continuously carrying all of that weight with her shoulders had made her back condition worse. She felt a touch of relief each weekend (the extra sleep might've helped) but by Monday morning she was hurting again and pining for her Friday appointment. All week long, as her bra straps bit into her shoulders, Laura was reminded of the source of her discomfort.

From high up in the bleachers where no one could detect the dejection on her face, Jennifer watched the girls on her high school basketball team celebrate another win. Part of her wanted to be back on the team with her friends, but thinking about being called "Jiggly Jenny" was even more painful than running up and down the court. Since freshman year, when her basketball skills began being compromised by her growing—and unsupported— chest, Jenny faced increasing flack for her changing physical appearance. As her breasts grew larger and she struggled to find the right bra to support them, even some of her teammates used the hated nickname. Jennifer was not only losing out on the chance to play basketball; she was losing her positive self-image.

Kate, Laura, and Jennifer have all suffered needlessly and prove that wearing the wrong bra can be hazardous to your health for many reasons. Whether it's too tight, too big, or just doesn't fit right, the consequences can be much more than merely physical. All women—and men, for that matter—connect their physical health with their emotional well-being. If our bodies feel good, we usually feel better about ourselves. But when we are in physical pain, our emotional welfare may be seriously challenged. Whether you're a teenager, a mother, or a career woman, you're entitled to feel good about yourself, free of any physical, emotional, or psychological handicaps that may be needlessly holding you back from enjoying life to its fullest.

Once Upon a Time, When Fit Was a Fairy Tale

To understand how wearing the right bra can affect your body and soul, it might help to know how this whole process began and how the history of fitting bras has evolved into what it is today.

Bra fitting can be confusing because there are so many pieces to literally fit together, and it's not something most American women are taught—not at home, in school, or anywhere else. There's no real mechanism for that education. Many mothers overlook the chance to help their daughters get fit correctly, perhaps because they never experienced the benefits of the right fit themselves. That leaves specialty stores, but some of them only offer a rudimentary fitting. Even the stores that do offer fittings drastically differ in the quality of the information they provide.

A comfortable, flattering, and healthy fit hasn't always been quite so challenging. Historically, stores employed professional fitters who helped women find their proper size. Before the Depression, each store housed foundation departments with a staff that routinely fit undergarments. Women purchased their brassieres utilizing sales personnel in higher quality department stores and specialty shops. Self-service was for low-end retailers only. An established fitting process existed in which a customer would go into the foundations department and explain her needs. Afterward, she was shown to a private fitting room to be measured and presented with appropriate options. Once choices were established, the foundation pieces were pinned and altered for a customized fit.

Department store managers or manufacturer's representatives trained the saleswomen to analyze a customer's figure and to fit her bra accordingly. The training programs were scientific and extensive, to the point that one manufacturer created a five-day course in fitting, complete with written final exams. Course graduates were awarded diplomas. Not only were the fitters educated; the stores went to great lengths to employ a range of women, varying in age and size, so that customers had someone similar in the fitting room with them. In those days, fitters had respected roles in the department store hierarchy, in part because store managers found that proper fit was good for the bottom line, which meant repeat customers and fewer returns.

But the realities of the Depression spelled doom for most retailers. Previous standards of personalized care went out the window, and it stayed that way for the next two decades. The habit of using fitters eventually saw its resurgence during the baby boom era, but it was short-lived. As the trend toward over-the-counter sales became more evident by the end of the 1950s, cost-saving policies meant that stores didn't want to pay the higher wages required to employ specialized, professional fitters.

As these valued employees left the stores, manufacturers began compensating for the lack of in-store, personal care by selling their bras in packaged boxes, complete with product information and fitting instructions. For the time being, this maintained a direct line of education from the manufacturers to its customers. But by the 1960s, racks of bras with little to no accompanying information could be seen on display in stores throughout America, leaving women to their own devices as far as sizing and fit were concerned.

Things aren't so different today, at least in your average department store. Even specialty shops that offer fit as a service vary widely when it comes to knowledge and training. The truth is, your fit will be only as good as your salesperson. Some of them may be great, while others are lacking, concentrating more on selling you the more profitable brands than what fits you best. That variability and questionable sense of priorities can lead to a lot of confusion about bra size.

According to Susan Nethero, founder of the Intimacy chain of high-end bra fit stores, "Eighty-five percent of women are wearing the wrong bra size and 65 percent of our customers have never had a fitting." It's time to change those numbers.

A Brief History of the Bra

Pre World War I
Women were bound by constricting corsets—as restrictive as their roles in society.

WWI
Women asked to stop buying corsets, in order to use the steel for producing warships.

The Roaring Twenties
Women gained independence and voting rights. Confining underwear made dancing impossible.

1931
Lastex, the revolutionary fiber, created the snap heard round the world, with its elastic core wound with fabric thread, creating two-way stretch for the first time.

World War II
Rosie the Riveter needed to be contained without being constrained; bras of the day did just that.

Post World War II
An hourglass figure became the feminine ideal, as modeled by Marilyn Monroe; the bullet bra became the norm.

1960s
Twiggy meant breasts were out and legs were in. Protesters at the 1968 Miss America Pageant didn't burn their bras. They threw them—along with mops, girdles, and Playboy magazines—into a trash can—but never actually torched it.

1970s
Women in the work force celebrated financial independence and a newly found sexual liberation. Bras become as

brightly colored and wild as a disco ball. Think *Charlie's Angels* jigglefest.

1980s

As power suits ruled the day, and women stormed the boardroom, out went the exhibitionism of the 70s.

1990s

The Wonderbra was introduced; curves were back, raising breast awareness to new heights.

2005

Oprah Winfrey's "Bra Intervention" shifted American thinking about what women wear under their clothes.

Today it's possible to find gorgeous bras in sizes ranging from 28AA to 56N.

Inventory Blues

Generally speaking, department stores stock bras with band sizes ranging from 32 to 38/40 and cup sizes in B to D/DD. While this range fits a large number of women, many fall outside of these parameters.

Why do stores maintain such a narrow assortment of sizes? For some, a limited inventory is due to cost. It's much less expensive to stock a limited size range because a bigger inventory needs more space. With that in mind, perhaps some store owners feel that larger sizes have less hanger appeal than smaller garments. Or stores may simply not want the responsibility of educating their employees about fitting a wider variety of body types and choose to simplify whatever bra-fitting education they offer.

All you really need to care about is going into a store and finding a bra that fits. Some women get so frustrated they will end up shoehorning themselves into a bra that's the wrong size, leaving them unsupported, uncomfortable, and unhealthy. But like you keep hearing in this book, it doesn't have to be that way!

Size Doesn't Mean Fit

Women may end up selecting the wrong bra simply because standards for fit vary from brand to brand, and sizes differ completely from country to country. In general, standards for size are consistent in cups B through D. However, the smallest cups and the larger sizes have no common international standards. In fact, the exact same bra may be called a DDD-cup in the United States, an E-cup in the United Kingdom, and an F-cup in France. If you're shopping in a store that imports bras (which most do) how are you supposed to tell the difference? With different brands labeling their bras with an assortment of names, how can you figure out your size?

No matter what is causing the confusion, the result is the same. So when you go bra shopping, forget about the names and the labels. Focus on how a bra fits your body.

To download your own International Cup Size Conversion Pocket Guide, go to www.fabfoundations.com/bustedextras

In chapter 6, you'll find an information box, comparing and contrasting different brands, both foreign and domestic. Below, you'll find an international cup size conversion chart. Both can be quite handy when bra shopping.

International Cup Size Conversion Chart

American	European	British	French	Italian	Australian
AAA	-	-	-	-	-
AA	AA	AA	-	-	-
A	A	A	A	A	A
B	B	B	B	B	B
C	C	C	C	C	C
D	D	D	D	D	D
DD/E	E	DD	E	DD	DD
DDD/F	F	E	F	E	E
DDDD/G	G	F	G	F	F
DDDDD/H	H	FF	H	-	FF
DDDDDD/I	-	G	J	-	G
J	-	GG	K	-	GG
K	-	H	-	-	H
L	-	HH	-	-	HH
M	-	J	-	-	J
N	-	JJ	-	-	JJ
-	-	K	-	-	-
-	-	L	-	-	-

The Hazards of Wearing the Wrong Bra

The physical consequences of poor bra fit include tension in your shoulders, upper back, neck, and head, or your upper body may become strained to a point that ultimately causes poor posture. If your bra band is too tight, you might get headaches or mistakenly put pressure on your lungs. If you carry the weight of your breasts in the bra straps, you can cause permanent divots in your shoulders.

Additional ill effects from wearing a poorly fit bra often include skin irritation, rashes, and infection from sweat and friction. For some women, these can become extremely uncomfortable. The most common side effects are the ones most women tend to fear the most, namely, sagging and vertical stretch marks.

Eveden, a British lingerie manufacturer, conducted field research and learned that 53 percent of women physically suffer from poor bra fit, and out of these, 24 percent would even consider plastic surgery to correct the damage.

The British Chiropractic Association has warned that "wearing the wrong bra size can lead to a number of problems, including back pain, restricted breathing, abrasions, breast pain and poor posture." Independent medical and scientific studies, both in the United Kingdom and in the States, have attested to the difficulties of getting the fit right and the implications of getting it wrong.

It's never too late to reconsider what bras you are wearing. Even women who think they've been fitted correctly and think they know their size are often wearing the wrong size. Since they don't understand fit for themselves, they have no idea that they are potentially harming their long-term health.

The Emotional Consequences

Problems with poor fit are not limited to physical symptoms. Manufacturers and store owners alike also report that poor bra fit can have direct emotional consequences.

Infomat, a leading market research company, conducted a study revealing that a badly fitted bra makes 59 percent of women feel more self-conscious. Their 2010 Intimates

Market Report states that "As women and men in America have been gaining weight, so too has their need to feel more sexy and desirable. Moreover, their self confidence has taken a hard nose dive."

Bra fit is about much more than just size or even comfort. As Sarah Wiener, owner of Trousseau in Vienna, Virginia, observes, "You're not really fitting just the bra, you're fitting a woman's self-image, her body image, and the societal perspective, and that comes with a lot of baggage."

Some women feel a sense of breast shame and that's reinforced by messages projected on a daily basis in the media. The small-busted may feel like less of a woman, almost as if they don't quite count because there's not enough breast to fill a cup.

Amanda Sage Barnum, blogger for 32aabra.com reports that, "When you can't even fill an A cup, it's like you don't exist as a woman."

Small-busted women have heard it all, like being told to shop in the children's department for training bras, or get implants, or they may have even been told that they don't need to wear a bra at all. That could make the less endowed feel like they're not even counted among the ranks of women.

Full-cupped ladies may end up feeling like they are too much woman, as if an overabundance is somehow unseemly. Some women have been told they should "cut em off." Because so many brands stop manufacturing at a DD-cup or smaller, many women have difficulty finding anything in commercial stores that fits. Some feel looked down upon, especially since they don't have the same option as small-busted sisters to go without.

All too often, women who are confident and successful in other realms of their lives walk into a dressing room carrying anger and insecurity.

Ellen Jacobson, president of the Elila brand, makes the following observation:

"Women often see themselves as the media wants them to, which makes buying or fitting the right bra such a challenge."

Ask Ali

Q: I get what you mean about the consequences of poor fit because I'm suffering from the works: back pain, stretch marks, and ache in my shoulders. I feel the bite of my bra every single day and it's depressing. How much of this is really reversible and how much of it is permanent?

Thanks,
Sophie,
Margate NJ

A: The majority of your issues can be gradually reversed. Back pain caused by an improperly fitting bra and divots on your shoulders can eventually be reduced and sometimes eliminated when you begin to wear bras that fit. (Before I found FabFit™, I had huge shoulder dents that are now barely visible.) That's the good news. On the flip side, once breast tissue is stretched, there's no way to undo it. Some women use creams for stretch marks, but honestly, the marks won't be fixed by wearing a better bra.

How to Lose Ten Pounds Without Going on a Diet

Beyond the physical problems associated with poor fit, an ill-fitting bra will make you look heavier in your clothes because your breasts will sit lower on your torso and mask the narrowest part of your rib cage. When the proper fit lifts your breasts, the thinner area of your rib cage is nicely exposed and that can leave you looking up to 10 pounds lighter—another welcome advantage.

The Right Bra Can Be Life Changing

No matter how uncomfortable you feel in your bra every day, and even if you've already experienced some of the physical or emotional problems associated with poor fit, it's never too late to start reversing the process. Finding a bra that fits properly is the first step to positive change. It's also a fabulous way to demonstrate how you value your own body.

Women who have gone through the FabFit™ process—particularly those who have had challenges finding bras that fit—consistently describe that process as a revelation. For some, it may seem farfetched to say that a small scrap of fabric can change a life. But finding proper bra fit is about more than the bra. The confidence that stems from knowing that you look your best is life changing.

"Once women find a bra that fits," says Amanda Sage Barnum, "they don't just talk about the bra; they say that they finally feel attractive."

How you feel is what The FabFit™ Formula is all about.

Size doesn't matter; it's the fit. It doesn't matter what size a bra is as long as it feels good, looks good, and doesn't need adjustment throughout the day. A great-fitting bra will make all the difference in how your clothes—and you—look and feel.

—Sarah Wiener, Owner, Trousseau, Vienna, Virginia

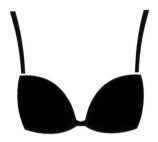

3

The Secret to Your Bra Size

ost bra measurement systems have a one-size-fits-all approach. Every woman, no matter what her size or shape may be, is given the same way to measure herself to determine what size bra will fit her best. But one size does NOT fit all!

As we've already learned, the concept of a woman's bra size was born on Madison Avenue in an advertising agency made up entirely of men. It didn't have its roots in real women's bodies, and unfortunately—no, unbelievably—it still exists today, complete with the same cup and band sizing problems that first existed decades ago.

Rather than continuing to wish for a different system, the best way to approach bra fit is to concentrate on making the existing process work for you in spite of its shortcomings. Once you understand how bra sizing really works you can use that knowledge to create your own FabFit™.

There's No Such Thing as Cup Size

One essential piece in the bra-fit equation is rarely explained to women, but it will unlock a key misunderstanding about the entire fitting process. Here it is:

Bra size is comprised of two components: the band and the cup.
They are not independent; they're interrelated.

As band size increases, the cup sewn onto that band increases, too. In other words, a B-cup on a 34 band is going to have an incrementally smaller cup than a B-cup on a 36 bra, and a larger cup in comparison to a 32B.

With each increase or decrease in band, the cup gets incrementally larger or smaller by one cup size. For example, the cup on a 34B is the same as a 32C or a 30D. This is why some stores will try to tell you that, for example, a 36C is the same as a 34D. The cup size is the same, but the way they support your body will be different. That margin becomes the difference between a bra that's just OK and one that truly fits.

The flip side of bra/cup interrelation is that it turns the idea of cup size on its head. The idea that you can say anybody is an "X-cup" is fundamentally flawed because cup size is irrelevant if you don't attach it to a correlated band size. A woman with a tiny rib cage could wear a 30DD and it would never match anyone's preconceived notion of what a DD-sized chest looks like, since the cups on a 30DD are the same size as on a 36B.

The Myth of the DD

Speaking of DD-cup bras, there are some serious myths out there about the women who fill these bras and their actual size. Most women have a tendency to focus on cup size alone to determine what is a large chest. People think of a DD-cup bra or a DD-cup woman as being huge, i.e., busty, busting out all over, and downright boobalicious. As we have just learned, that is a major misconception, which leads people to confuse or simply ignore the relationship between the band and the cup. That basic misunderstanding leads many women astray.

Women and men alike buy into another myth of the DD, which is that bra sizes stop at that particular cup size. It's often true that most of the familiar places we shop may stop stocking bras at a DD-cup, which is probably why so many American women believe that DD represents the largest bra size. In fact, statistics show that 36DD is currently America's *average* bra size. (More on that in a minute.)

One final aspect of the myth of the DD is that anyone larger than a DD-cup must have a correspondingly large body — or is employed in the adult entertainment field—or both. That's silly and simply not true. Many leading bra manufacturers make bras in sizes like 28J and sell them to women with natural breasts. You can absolutely have a small rib cage and large breasts.

So, let's throw out the myth of the DD and focus on what's real.

Ask Ali

Q: I recently took my 17-year-old daughter to a store for a bra fitting and they told her she was a 32G. I had no idea that bras were even made in that size and I'm not sure what to do about it.
Does she need a breast reduction?

Best regards,
Penny, Lincoln, NE

A: Please don't rush a teenager into a breast reduction, even if she is uncomfortable with her breasts. Your daughter's body is still developing, and she may want the chance to make this irreversible decision for herself. Wearing quality bras that fit will keep your daughter supported and comfortable, which will play a significant role in what she decides to do. While a G-cup may seem large to you, your daughter will benefit most from finding the right bra for her, and feeling reassured that you love her and respect her for exactly who she is. In my experience, supporting a positive self-image will be more beneficial than any surgery.

Why Women's Bodies Are Changing

Women often misunderstand fit because of overall changes in women's bodies that have occurred over the past few decades. In the bra department, the average size in the 1970s was a 34B, but that has grown gradually and steadily bigger in both band and cup. Most Americans are shocked to learn that today's average bra size is a 36DD. They are further surprised to learn that bras are available in sizes ranging from 28 to 56 and cups that go from AAA to an N. Yes, N, like Nancy. In lingerie stores across the country, the need for larger sizes—beyond those found in most mainstream stores— is becoming more and more evident. As Susan Nethero, founder of the Intimacy chain of high-end lingerie stores, explains, "Seventy-four percent of my business is now at cup sizes larger than DD."

Why all the growth? Why are women's bodies changing so much?

There is no single scientific explanation. One possible answer is that the average overall body size in America, which is only getting bigger, is redefining the meaning of "average." This is not limited to women by any stretch of the imagination, but it does present particular problems for women searching for the right bra to fit their bodies.

Increasing breast size can be tied to the increasing amount of hormones that are being used in the commercial milk and meat we ingest as part of our regular diet. Many scientists view hormones as a major factor in the earlier onset age of puberty in girls. When development is increasingly seen beginning in pre-adolescent girls, it should come as no surprise that their breasts, growing for longer periods of time, end up becoming larger.

Some lingerie experts even suggest that vanity sizing in bras may play a role in the increased average bra size. The argument is that women's bodies have not actually changed. Rather, manufacturers are adjusting bra sizing toward smaller bands and larger cup sizes to make women feel better about themselves. The vanity sizing argument suggests that the average size is determined more as a result of marketing than biology. Even if vanity sizing does exist, it is simply further support for the theory that when it comes to bra purchases, it's the fit that matters, not the size. There's just no way to measure boobalicious.

All Fittings Are NOT Created Equal

The seemingly obvious course of action would be to go to the nearest store and get fitted for a bra. Sadly, there are relatively few stores that focus on fitting, and even when women are offered a fitting it's not always a good one. Not all stores that offer bra sizing as part of their mission have the ability to train and educate each individual member of their sales team, so the person who is helping you on a given day may or may not be talented at measuring, even in a store that has a reputation for fitting everyone. Factor in the number of stores that sell on commission, and there can be even more women ending up with bras that don't fit quite right. This is particularly true in the larger and smaller cup sizes: A-cup and below, or DD-cup and beyond.

Which? magazine, a British equivalent of *Consumer Reports*, investigated bra sizing in major stores throughout the United Kingdom. They used 11 researchers, ages 25 to 75, each with a DD cup size or larger, and met 70 different specialists in local stores while attempting to buy an everyday bra.

Some women were sold wildly different sizes by different shops. In one case, recommendations varied by seven sizes, from a 34FF to a 40D. Another researcher was sold exactly the same bra in two different stores, but in sizes 34C and 34F, both of which were a terrible fit. In another episode, despite their differences in age and body shape, a

30-year-old and a 75-year-old were sold the same push-up bra but it didn't fit either one of them.

We can conclude that even when women are going to specialized stores that measure for size, they will not always get a proper bra fit.

To download pocket shopping guides, handy charts, and other surprises, visit www.fabfoundations.com/bustedextras

Don't Let a Good Fitter Get Away

Of course there are great fitters out there in the United Kingdom and in the United States—incredibly knowledgeable, well-trained women who work in stores of all kinds. The fact is, a professional fitter can be your best friend when bra shopping. Any time you have a chance to get fitted by a professional—take it. A great fitter can help you find not only the sizes that work best for you, but also the styles and shapes that will highlight your figure to its best advantage.

In case you don't have the opportunity to work with someone wonderful, it's important to understand fit for yourself, but the value of working with a quality fitting professional cannot be underestimated.

Shopping for bras is somewhat like shopping for shoes: some brands run large or small, some run narrow or wide, and when you get into international sizes, sometimes there is little correlation. Also, like shoes, when shopping for bras you'll find that some brands or styles just fit you better. Each bra design is different, even within the same brand. Where your breasts sit on your chest and how you carry your tissue all factor into how a bra will fit you. There's just no way to know by looking at the label.

You have to try on a bra to know how it works for you.

Certain variables will have to be matched up with your personal preferences, for example, the amount of lift your bra provides, or the shape it gives your breasts. Other aspects of bra fit, are more objective, and these are the ones that will be covered in the rest of the book. Of all of the fit factors, most important is your understanding of the four key elements that determine how a bra will work on your body: band, cups, bridge, and straps.

FabFit™ is a formula, but beyond the mechanics, fit also requires the right state of mind. Let's call it a philosophy or, in this case, a Filosofy.

The Fab Fit™ Filosofy

Try on a bra to know how it fits YOU.
Remember: you don't have a size.
No measuring required!

Women of every size and shape have difficulty finding bras that fit, but once you learn how to meet that challenge you will look and feel better than ever. In the next chapter, we will break down how to fit your bra—step-by-step.

But first, take a minute to look in the back of the book and familiarize yourself with the Glossary and Guide to Bra Styles. Understanding the lingo will help you through the information being covered in chapter 4 and beyond.

Making something pretty is easy. Making something fit is hard. Women walk into a fitting room with a lot of anger and insecurity. That is such a challenge. It's emotional, behavioral and physical. And complicated. If it were easy, every woman would have a good fit.

—Ellen Jacobson, President, Elila

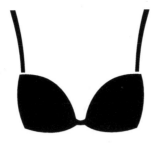

4

Fitting the Girls

In order to find your best bra fit and achieve the look you want, it helps to identify your specific personal preferences: the amount of lift your bra provides, the shape it gives your breasts, and how it works with your style of dress. All of these factors play a role in fashioning your overall fit. But no matter what your particular style may be, comfort and fit will always be your most important considerations.

The Bra Band

Your bra band is the most critical component in creating the optimal fit. The band should provide 80 to 90 percent of the support your breasts need. The goal is to achieve a fit that is firm, anchored, and horizontal. What do those words actually mean?

Firm: The band needs to be snug to your body and may feel tighter than what you are used to wearing. While you need that firmness for a proper fit, it should not feel uncomfortable when you breathe. The most common bra-fit error made by American women is a band that is too loose.

There are two ways to determine if your band is appropriately firm. You should be able to get only one or two fingers between the band and your skin. When you pull the band away from your body, it should have immediate resistance and should come only one inch (at most two) away from your body.

Anchored: When a bra band is anchored, it stays in place without riding up. You want your band to stay in the same position, whether you are putting your arms over your head, shifting your purse, carrying your groceries, lifting your laptop, or putting your luggage into an overhead bin. A properly fitting bra will stay in the same place on your back throughout your daily activities.

Horizontal: The horizontal position is circular, parallel to the floor, and lines up with the underside of your breasts, where they meet your rib cage. This position corresponds to the narrowest part of your torso, so once your bra is firmly anchored in the horizontal position, it should stay there.

You'll know your band is firmly anchored when it remains in a horizontal position on your back throughout the day. When you make the common error of using a band that is too loose, you'll notice that the band moves on your body or it lifts up in the back with normal movement.

For FabFit™ tips and tricks, go to
www.fabfoundations.com/bustedextras

The way to know if your band is, in fact, slipping is to look in the mirror after you've been wearing the bra for a few hours. Is the band in the same place you put it at the beginning of the day?

Here's an exercise to do in the morning, when you put on your bra in the horizontal position: With a pen, make a small mark in the middle of your back. Check it throughout the day. Is your bra still in the same place? If it's not, you're not firm, anchored, and horizontal.

Think of your bra as the seesaw on a children's playground. When the band comes up, the breasts go down. A firm, anchored, and horizontal band will lift your breasts.

The fibers on the band of a new bra may be fairly stiff and will begin to flex with a first wearing, so ensuring a firm, anchored, and horizontal fit from the outset is crucial.

That Dreaded Back Fat

Some women choose to wear a looser bra because they want to avoid that dreaded back fat. In fact, when your band is firm, anchored, and horizontal, it will create the smallest amount of visible lump in your back tissue.

This may seem counterintuitive, but part of the reason women get back fat is because their band is too loose. As the band rides up, it pushes the back flesh up over the course of the day, creating lumps. A back band that is too narrow can also create back fat by cutting into the skin on your back. That said, some women are just softer than others.

Following The FabFit™ Formula will minimize whatever back fat may be visible and may even eliminate it. It will also make you more comfortable and less bothered by any remaining lumps.

Is it a magic bullet? Not always, but it does provide your best chance for feeling as smooth as possible.

In order for a bra to do its job, it must adequately support your breasts. The wider the band, the more support. A wider band can also help to smooth the skin of the back. A band that is too thin can cut into the flesh, creating unsightly bra lines.

This doesn't mean that wider is better. A wider band will provide more stability, but it's also possible to have too much band for your body. For example, if your back is toned, it may not be accentuated by using a wider band.

Full-figured women generally need a wider band, but numbers can be deceiving. A 38 band can be worn by somebody who is soft, or it could be appropriate for an athlete with a muscular back. As with all things, the right fit for you is unique, and the focus should be on how the fit will enhance your body to its best advantage. It's important to assess your individual needs to find a band that will be firm, anchored, and horizontal.

Ask Ali

Q: I'm trying to figure out this firm, anchored, and horizontal thing. Right now, my band is making red marks on my body. Does that mean it's too tight?

Maria
Houston TX

A: Just because you get some red marks doesn't automatically mean a bra band is too tight. Even new socks can make a mark. A few things to check:

1. *The marks should fade quickly after removing your bra.*

2. *Make sure there's some give in your band, according to The FabFit™Formula.*

3. *Your bra should always be comfortable.*

A good bra is meant to provide support for the weight of your breasts, and distributing that weight correctly is important. Your band should carry 80 to 90 percent of your breast weight. Many women put too much stress on the straps, which leads to the physical issues discussed in chapter 2, such as shoulder aches, backaches, and shoulder divots.

Proper band fit addresses much of the weight distribution issue. Another thing to look for is the make-up of the band itself. A quality band has little stretch, and that will help keep it anchored. When a band is very stretchy, it's too easy for it to give way to the movements that are a part of everyday life, and it will not stay anchored on your back.

It's imperative that large-breasted women find bras with less stretch. You really want something that's going to fit snugly to the body, offering the support you need.

The Cup

A properly fitted cup keeps all of your breast tissue contained and shaped with nothing spilling out of the form defined by the design of the bra. The two easiest ways to spot an incorrect fit in the cup are quadboob and underspill.

Quadboob exists when the line of the bra cuts into your breast tissue, creating the illusion of four breasts, with two resting in the cups, and two spilling over the top, like islands cut off from the mainland. The effect is unsightly, easy to detect, and leaves your breasts bisected by the line of your cup. Ouch!

Having part of your bust spilling beneath the bottom of your cup is underspill. It's less obvious in your clothes, but can lead to rash and irritation under your breasts.

And because your breasts are not in the cup, they are not getting their needed support.

How can you tell if you have underspill? Lift your arms up and really move them around. If the bra pulls away from your body when you raise your arms and you can see any portion of the bottom of your breast, then you have underspill.

When you're looking at whether or not a cup is the right size for you, focus on the area behind the under-wire to ensure that it's capturing all the breast tissue. In other words, think of the underwire like a smile. All of the points below the smile are "behind" or "below" the underwire. As you feel below the underwire you should feel only bone and hard tissue; you should not feel any breast tissue. Breast tissue extends all the way under your arm, so even under the armpit the bra should encompass all of the soft tissue. When you capture all of that tissue in the cup, and the flesh under your band feels consistent as you press from the underwire toward your back, that is when your cup fits.

The shape of your bra cup has a lot to do with fit. A full-cup bra captures your entire breast, whereas a demi-cup, as the name suggests, covers only about half of it. If the bra doesn't fit just right, whatever you're wearing won't look so good, either. You want a smooth transition from the cup to your skin, without creating lines or bulges when you move. So if the cup cuts into your breast when you move around, then either the cup size or that particular style of bra may not be right for you.

While style is important, the materials used in the cups provide clues about how that bra will work. More rigid materials create a higher shape that aggressively alters your breasts, whereas something stretchy provides less structure. Some bras are cut into a rounder silhouette, while others create a more pointed effect. It's all personal preference. Some women prefer to sit higher; others don't want their breasts pushed up quite as far. Some like a rounder shape; some may wish to usher in a new era of the bullet bra. Knowing what you want will help guide you in the fitting room.

Are Your Cups Too Big or Too Small?

Determining whether your cups fit properly can make a big difference. Here are some clues to help you figure it out.

If your cups pucker or gap, that indicates that you have too much material in the cup and not enough bust to fill it, meaning, your cup is too big. Your body should fill the entire cup, beginning right at the underwire. If there is any gap between where the underwire ends and your breast begins, that's a further indicator of improper cup fit. On the flipside, bulges suggest a too-small cup. Your breast should not spill over, under, or out the sides of your cups.

One symptom of too-small cup size is when the center panel, or bridge, tips forward. Getting the bridge to sit correctly is an essential part of The FabFit™ Formula.

For some women, no matter how many cup styles they try, an underwire is simply not comfortable. If you're one of those women, a soft-cup bra may be the solution. For soft-cup bras, the fit of the band and cup follow the same formula. The biggest difference will be in the fit of the bridge.

The Bridge

The bridge is the centerpiece of the bra. Sometimes called the gore or the saddle, the bridge is the part of the bra that connects the two cups in the center. In an underwire bra, the bridge is a clear indicator of whether or not the bra is fitting properly. In a properly fitting underwire bra, the bridge should tack against your breastbone. In other words, it should lay flat against your skin in the middle between your breasts. It's only in very rare cases that a woman cannot find a bra to tack properly to her chest wall.

At this point, many of you may be saying, "I must be one of those rare cases."

You're probably not, unless you are in a cup size beyond what is manufactured for underwire bras. These days, underwire bras are manufactured in sizes up to an L cup. Many women insist that they can't get the gore to tack, until they find a different style, which actually works for them. In other words, if the gore of your underwire bra doesn't tack, the problem is most likely with the fit of your bra, not your body.

Some women have concave chests, meaning that the space between their breasts is actually sunken compared to the rest of their chest wall. For those women, it is also a challenge to get the gore to tack.

Frederika Zappé, national fit specialist for the Eveden brands (including Freya, Fantasie, and Elomi), recommends the narrowest possible gore for customers with a concave chest. The lower the gore, she says, the more the chest wall can be removed from the bra-fit equation. One may not be able to find a bra that tacks perfectly, but a shallower gore will do its best to create an ideal fit.

The above is true only for underwire bras. If you're wearing a soft-cup bra, you're not necessarily going to be able to get the bridge to tack because, by design, the cups on these bras have to sit much higher on your chest in order to provide the same support as an underwire bra. Bridge tacking refers primarily to underwire bras. If you're a soft-cup fan, don't ignore the gore. Try to minimize the gap for your own FabFit™.

When evaluating whether a bra style will work for you, think in terms of whether your own breasts sit narrower or wider on your chest wall. How you carry your bust needs to match up with the style of the bra you select, and one way of improving your fit is to choose a garment with a bridge whose width corresponds to your body type.

Many brands change the size of the bridge with the cup size. The larger the cup size, the closer together those cups sit on the bra, but not all styles are cut the same. Look for a bra that best matches what you need for your unique body.

But what about women who insist that they "carry wide?" Oftentimes, that's simply bra-fitter code for improper fit. If your band is too loose and your cup is too small, it's easy to feel like you carry wide. Use The FabFit™ Formula and look for styles that work with your body for the best results.

The Straps

The straps of your bra need to be firm while not digging into your shoulders. Since 80 to 90 percent of the support in your bra should come from the band, that leaves only 10 to 20 percent coming from the straps.

The straps should be comfortable. Too often, women try to add lift to their breasts by over-tightening the straps. Breasts can be heavy, and if the majority of that weight is resting on your shoulders all day, you will end up with a fair amount of discomfort and stress. Over time, other health problems will probably accumulate.

Remember Anita, whose bra straps constantly slipped off her shoulders? That's not uncommon. Tightening the straps would seem to be the obvious solution. But while straps get the blame, they aren't always the culprit. Sometimes, falling straps indicate improper fit. Perhaps the straps are set too wide for your shoulders. Or your cup size may be too big and not suited to your breast shape. Straps can also slip when your band is too big and rides up, leaving too much play in the straps.

If you have narrow shoulders or suffer from strap slippage, look for strap styles that are set closer to the center of the cup or are attached closer to the middle of the band in the back—or both.

Understanding Your Underwire

If your underwire is poking you in the armpit, it may be because of the bra you've selected, or perhaps your body is short in the torso. Either way, it's a miserable way to go through your day. To remedy, take another look at the bra you're wearing. Each design is slightly different, and there may be another brand or style that is lower under the arm. Some high-end boutiques will even alter the underwire to fit you, but start by seeing if there's another bra style that works better for you.

Sometimes women notice that their underwire is cutting into their breast tissue, and that's a different problem. That's a fit issue, and an indicator of a cup that's too small. The worst underwire problems occur when the wire breaks free and begins poking through your bra prematurely. Not only is it uncomfortable, a lot of times that's actually a sign of improper fit. Specifically, a band that's too large can move around too much on your body, ultimately allowing the underwire to wear through its housing. Any time your band isn't anchored, it rubs against your body, creating friction that can wear down the bra's fibers.

How the Bra Should Fit YOU

Bra fitting is very personal, which is why it's so difficult—no, impossible—to have a one-size-fits-all approach. For example, some women, like opera singers or athletes, have rib cages that expand more than others when they take a deep breath.

These women may need more room in the band because their chest simply expands more than average when they breathe deeply. No matter what your lifestyle may be, your bra needs to accommodate your natural daily routine.

Understanding how your band, cups, bridge, and straps should fit is extremely important. But it's not the whole picture. The next step in The FabFit™ Formula involves a focus on how a bra will fit your unique body shape. This combination of skills is the heart of FabFit™ and is essential for being comfortable in your bra. Even more, it's an important element for looking and feeling amazing, both physically and mentally.

Many women are okay with their bodies but shopping makes them feel like they are wrong. Some women have the same measurement but different dimensions. Even within cup sizes, there's a range of plus/minus. You have to know the bras and how they look on a person's body. Women are crying because they are so beaten up, like there's something wrong with them. A woman wants to be able to choose, to feel like a woman.

—Ellen Shing, Lula Lu, San Francisco

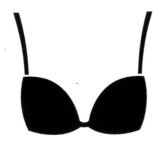

5

Which Body Type Are You?

When it comes to bras, your body type falls into one of four major groups: petite, standard, full-busted, and full-figured. Identifying your particular category is essential to finding your best bra fit. That also applies to bra styles. Each body type—and bra style—has its own particular characteristics and, happily, each one offers gorgeous bras that will make you look and feel—Fab.

Petite

"Petite" has a different definition in lingerie than it does in clothing. In lingerie, a petite woman is one with a smaller bust. It's not height or weight related. There was a time when petite lingerie had a narrower definition, including both a small rib cage and cup size. Recently, the clamour from women with a larger rib cage (up to a 48 band) combined with a small cup size has led to an expanded definition of petite, and manufacturers have provided more options accordingly.

Regardless of size, every woman should be wearing a bra. It's not a question of appearance or modesty. Keeping breast tissue properly supported is a matter of good health. While it may feel great to go braless in your twenties, you can do irreversible damage to the ligaments in your breasts if you go without proper support. Over time, that will lead to more sagging, even for those with the smallest busts.

When bra shopping, petite women have their own issues, usually on the opposite end of the spectrum from their bustier sisters; namely, they tend to wear a bra that is too small in the band and too large in the cup. This stems from the relationship between band and cup size.

A woman who might be a 36AA could end up wearing a 34A or even a 32B because she can't find stores that stock her size. The smaller size band will be her only option since the cup size on the 36AA, the 34A, and the 32B will all be roughly equivalent. But wearing a band that's several inches too small will be extremely uncomfortable.

For petite women, even a 32A bra may not wrap around the body properly because a woman may not fit neatly into a bra that is essentially a scaled-down version of a standard size. That's one reason why there's been an increased number of manufacturers catering specifically to the petite bra market. These specialized brands are doing their best to address a petite woman's unique needs.

Small breasts also don't always mean a narrow position on the rib cage. Breasts don't grow closer together just because they're smaller. In fact, small-busted women can have breasts quite wide apart. Mainstream cups tend to be too deep and positioned too close together when compared to bras that are developed specifically for a petite body.

Feeling Good About Petite

Many petite women are quite okay with their bodies, but once they go bra shopping they start feeling insecure. While women who wear a petite bra size may have bodies with similar measurements as girls wearing a training bra, the difference in the mindset of the target customer can be huge. What a mature woman with a petite body wants in a bra often differs from what a young girl may be looking for in her first bra. Sexy and lacy can be fantastic attributes in a bra but they are not necessarily appropriate for a pre-teen.

Petite women find it embarrassing to be sent to the children's section or told that they don't need to wear a bra. For Christina, who you met in chapter 1, being told to shop in the children's department was beyond humiliating; it cut to the essence of her feelings about being a woman, and every time Christina was told she didn't need a bra, that feeling resurfaced.

Every woman wants to feel feminine and have choices when it comes to how she expresses herself. She also wants to look professional. For example, just because you're small busted, doesn't mean you're small nippled, and it can look and feel awkward for a petite woman operating in the business world when she feels like her nipples are showing.

Since petite bras are so seldom stocked in an average store, women who need them may not have found a bra that fits correctly and highlights their body's assets. That can seriously compromise how customers in the petite market feel about themselves. Many say they never felt like a real woman before finding an authentic petite bra.

Emily Lau, the owner of The Little Bra Company, a petite bra manufacturer, has observed many women being correctly fitted for the first time. She reports that, "they can become emotional, saying, 'that's what I'm supposed to look like.'"

Within the petite bra market, some manufacturers focus on designs that enhance what nature has given you, with padding specifically designed to push existing tissue up and in. Other companies choose to celebrate your natural size, without enhancement. These options represent nothing more than personal preference and are a reflection of the greater number of bras being designed for petite frames.

Specific bra styles may look better on a petite-busted body. It helps to use all the breast tissue she can, for example, if a woman has less tissue on the top of her breast. In other words, if the majority of her tissue is below her nipple, then a demi bra may be a good option. If a woman carries fuller or higher, then a T-shirt or a balcony bra might be a better choice. A plunge bra pushes everything from the side forward, which can be great for low-cut tops. If you carry wider, you may not have enough breast tissue to create cleavage.

In any case, petite women ultimately want the same thing as any other woman: the chance to look and feel great, and to develop a positive self-image.

Standard

Standard sizes are essentially in the range of a 32 to 38 band and a B to D cup. In other words, these are the sizes that are typically found in most major stores.

For those who can't easily find bras in commercial stores, it may seem like women wearing standard sizes have it made, enjoying the luxury of going into any local store to shop for a bra. But just because women who fall into the standard category have easy access to bras, it doesn't mean they're getting properly fitted. In fact, there is no evidence to suggest that women who wear standard-size bras do any better than petite or busty women when it comes to fit.

Women of standard sizes must undergo the same process to determine the back, cup, bridge, and strap combinations that work best for them. Like everyone else, how you carry your breasts will determine the bra style that offers the best shape.

Breasts that need more support may select full and balconette styles, while perkier and wide-set breasts will work well in demi-cup shapes. Contour-cup styles are popular in this size range as well. This smooth, shaped-cup style does a great job for a seamless look, nipple control, and evening out asymmetry.

Fit challenges exist in every size and body type, so it's equally important for women in the standard-size range to assess their FabFit™ Formula.

Are You Uneven?

Bra shopping can be particuarly challenging for women with breasts that are noticeably uneven in size, otherwise known as having asymmetrical breasts. While almost all women have some breast asymmetry, up to 25 percent of women are visibly uneven, which means a difference of at least one cup size. Ten percent of you are more than one cup size apart.

So how do you fit yourself?

You always fit the larger breast, and if necessary, use some kind of padding to even things out in the smaller cup. Try formed or contour cups to provide the illusion of more symmetry.

Having your best bra fit—and the knowledge that being uneven is very common— may help aleviate the insecurity some women feel about having asymmetrical breasts.

Full-Busted

If you have a band size 38 or smaller, and a cup size DD or larger, then you are considered to be full-busted. There are brands that cater expressly to this body type, with band sizes that begin at 28 and cup sizes that go as high as an L-cup.

As full-busted women, you face different fit challenges compared to petite or standard women. There can be a misconception that larger busts sit on correspondingly larger bodies, so finding stores that carry your size can be a challenge. Most full-busted women tend to wear a band that's too big and cups that are too small. This may be because so many shops stock only up to a DD-cup.

For example, let's say a woman's best fit will be in a 34F bra. When she goes into a store with the standard range of sizes, a 34DD won't begin to fit her breasts. If she doesn't even know that bras exist in sizes beyond a DD-cup, maybe she will choose a 36 or 38 band bra because the corresponding DD will have a larger cup.

But will it really fit?

Any time you wear a bra with a band that's too big, you will not get the firm, anchored, and horizontal foundation you need to achieve proper fit. As covered in chapter 2, larger breasts that go consistently under-supported are at risk of getting irreversible, vertical stretch marks. The physical effects of poor fit can begin with simple discomfort and skin irritation and go so far as to cause the shape of your body to change as it accommodates the weight of your breasts sitting on your shoulders.

As a full-busted woman, you want bras with adequately supporting back bands. Something too narrow will not provide the support your body requires. That doesn't mean you have to wear an unattractive bra. There are plenty of gorgeous, lacy, sexy bras in your size, as well as attractive, conservative, functional styles. No matter what your taste, there are many styles to choose from, when you know where to look.

For the full-busted woman, a lingerie store offering a wide range of sizes will be your best option to ascertain which bras suit you best. If there's no store near you with adequate selection, go to www.fabfoundation.com/bust-edextras for FabFit™ internet shopping support.

The shape of your breast determines your best fit. For a busty woman, a demi-cup bra is not often as supportive unless you are very firm and high and carry less flesh on the top side of your breast. Some manufacturers have recently begun making quasi-demi cups, with more structure, enabling full-busted women access to the sexy demi-cup look without sacrificing fit. A cut and sewn bra—seamed with several panels—is a good option for full-busted and full-figured women. The rule of thumb is, the more seams in a bra, the more support. Full-cup and balconette styles are often good options for the full-busted.

Molded bras are more challenging to fit in fuller sizes because body and breast shapes differ increasingly as they get larger. It may also be difficult to find strapless styles at the larger end of the cup spectrum, particularly above an H-cup, although manufacturers continue to expand their lines. Another way for the full-busted to get great strapless support is in a long-line bra, which provides support by extending fabric further down the torso.

Full-Figured

The full-figured woman has a band size that starts at around a 38-band with a cup size above a DD. In truth, there are no exact measurements to define full-figured because it has so much to do with each individual's body.

Full-figured women tend to wear a band that's too big and a cup that's too small, much for the same reasons as the full-busted woman. The difference between a full-figured and a full-busted woman has to do with the amount of construction required to do the job of supporting the bust. A full-figured woman may need something more constructed in order to achieve her best bra fit.

Because shoulders don't necessarily increase proportionally with body size, bra straps can tend to slip off more easily for full-figured women, particularly when narrow shoulders are added to the mix. You want to look for a bra style with a strap that comes from the center of the cup, rather than a wide-set strap, to reduce the possibility of slipping. A trend with current bra styles is a wider-set strap, which can be a great look under clothes, but it's not going to serve you well if your bra strap is constantly slipping off your shoulder.

Full-figured women may also seek out thicker straps, in order to distribute the weight of the chest over a wider area of the shoulder. Even with the band doing the majority of the work, it's still important to minimize the weight digging into any one point on the shoulder.

The number of rows of clasps on a band, known as hooks and eyes, can make a difference in the amount of support a bra provides, with at least three rows suggested for full-figured women. Additional padding around the underwire can help the comfort level, and extra support, such as side stays (small boning in the band) all help enhance excellent fit for full-figured women. The more support you need, the more important it is to have a firm fit in the band.

Some women who have more meat on their bones may still have softness underneath the band that's not breast tissue. If your body has some extra padding and you're not sure if you are capturing all of the breast tissue when testing the fit of your cup, try prodding the area underneath the bra band. The amount of flesh you notice under the band should feel the same all the way up to the underwire.

If you're short-waisted and full-busted, you have one of the most challenging body types to fit. You may have trouble finding a bra that will encase the bust on the chest wall, because proportionately there's not enough support. Fortunately, some manufacturers are designing bras expressly for your body type. These are bandless in the front, meaning the bottom of the underwire is the end of the bra, with no band beneath the underwire. These are good for full-figured, short-waisted women because the bras minimize the amount of structure between the bottom of the breast and the waist.

Notes to All Large-Breasted Ladies

Large breasts need somewhere to sit. In order to get the bridge to tack to your body for optimal support, you may need to focus on styles that will accommodate your fuller breasts. A lot of full-busted women have trouble getting the bridge to tack, and many insist that it's impossible to get it to adhere to the chest wall, claiming there is no room for a bridge to wedge in between their breasts. Fear not. There is a bra out there for virtually everybody. It just may take a little longer to find it.

If you have trouble getting the bridge to tack, try looking for bras that have a narrower or shorter bridge, with less material attaching the cups together. Less bridge means there is less fabric that needs to stay tacked against your body. That narrower bridge will give your breasts more room to sit, while also allowing your bra to tack to your breastbone. This is particularly true if your breasts are very round or quite close together—or both.

Full-busted and full-figured women should look for bras that add mesh and other stretch-resistant fabrics to the bands to improve that firm fit. It's worth saying again: getting the band to fit correctly is necessary for your FabFit™.

Busting the Myth of the Minimizer

Many large-busted women are encouraged to try minimizer bras. In theory, a minimizer bra makes you look up to one cup size smaller, which helps women who prefer to de-emphasize their breasts or help them fit more easily into their clothes. Minimizers work if you're eyeing your body from its profile. But how do they work?

Most minimizers redistribute breast tissue, spreading it out while pushing it against the chest wall. While the profile of the breast is minimized, the breasts end up looking lower and wider. Minimizers are favored bras by many women and can provide a good fit. But minimizers, because of their design, may end up making your overall figure appear lower and wider, which you may not like.

For more body type information and extra features, visit www.fabfoundations.com/bustedextras.

The Grass is Always Greener

No matter what your body type, it's common for women to think that the grass is always greener on the other side of the fence when it comes to breast size.

At one fitting, a busty woman came into the dressing room wearing a sports bra. It was the only kind of bra she wore, because she didn't like her curves and the sports bra made her feel smaller. But the effect was not flattering – the bra smashed her breasts against her body. Like an extreme minimizer, the sports bra made her bust profile lower, but her entire breast was wider on her body. It masked her figure, so when she was fitted properly, the effect was dramatic. She, literally, squealed with delight, exclaiming, "I look tiny! I barely even recognize myself, I look so small!"

In another instance, a woman came in for a fitting wearing a bra that was stretched out and sagging. She laughingly shared that it was a ten year-old bra, one from the days before she'd had children. Needless to say, her body had seen some changes, and the 36B garment no longer did the trick. The fitting revealed that she should, in fact, be wearing a 32DD. From the dressing room, she called her husband to share the news – it's unclear which of them was more thrilled with her new size.

It just goes to show, across the board, women of every breast size get their fit wrong and share similar insecurities when it comes to both bra shopping and their bodies.

No matter what your body size or shape may be, the steps for fit are the same. Assess your band, cup, bridge, and straps, taking into account your individual body type. The more in touch you are with what works best for you, the more successful you will be when it comes to fitting your unique body.

At the end of the day, even if you have a great fitter in the dressing room, you know your body better than anyone else. Your best FabFit™ means looking better, feeling better, and getting the most value from your bras.

When the material is less good quality it won't last as long. It won't retain its shape. The fibers break down. The underwires are more likely to pop out. There's a disposable mentality.

—Layla L'Obatti, Designer, Between The Sheets

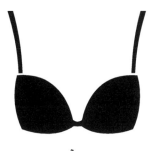

6

Your Best Bra for the Buck

*N*ow that you've learned about size and fitting and have identified your body type, it's almost time to go shopping. But before we send you off to purchase your dream bra, it's essential that you understand more about how a bra is constructed and how costs vary.

A bra is a complex piece of clothing, probably more than any other item in your wardrobe. A high-quality bra can often have 38—and even as many as 55—individual pieces. On a manufacturing floor, 25 different people can touch a single bra as it moves down the line. When you think about what you're asking of your bra, especially in larger cup sizes, it's amazing what that little bit of fabric can do.

Bra Innovations

Today's bras contain a surprising amount of technological innovation.

Take the spacer bra, for example, a new material used in some contour-cup bras. The cups have air built in between its two layers of fabric. Because spacer bras have the ability to move more freely than other contour bras, they offer less gapping in the cup, as they adhere to fit your individual breast shape.

Spacer bras are generally made with a more rigid back band to account for their flexible shape in the front. Keep in mind that flexible doesn't necessarily mean stretchy; it's still a firm fit.

Another nifty innovation particularly good for women is a heat transferring, cool fabric, patented by Amoena. The fabric actually transfers heat to and from the body, which is helpful for women with implants, prostheses, and those affected by irritation under their breasts.

"By incorporating Comfort+, the bra literally pulls heat away from the body to reduce perspiration," says Lesley Pfitzenmayer, Development Manager of Amoena's textile design team.

Why Some Bras Are More Expensive Than Others

There is generally a correlation between the complexity of a garment and its price. Some factors that can drive up the cost of a bra are engineering, construction, fabric, embellishments, and hand sewing. When you understand what you're paying for, you can make a more informed selection.

Engineering and Construction

Every bra goes through a design process. The highest quality bras use that process to ensure an excellent fit with every size they offer. Engineering is part of design; it's the aspect that ensures a bra will do its job of supporting the breast, all while looking good.

Simply put, the bigger your cup size, the more your bra needs engineering. For example, look at the straps. They should not stretch too much while still staying firmly attached to the rest of the bra. The rings to adjust the straps should be made out of strong material, like durable plastic or metal. Any bras with thin, bendable, plastic adjusters won't provide a stable fit and will wear out quickly.

The amount of stretch in the straps can be an indicator of quality. Empreinte, a luxury French brand, engineers a reduced degree of elasticity in the straps of its bras—30 percent versus 50 percent for a standard strap—creating much firmer support. That being said, you don't want to eliminate stretch. Some elasticity is necessary to achieve a fit that moves with your body throughout the day.

Engineering can be less visible to consumers. For example, most people don't realize that some British manufacturers use specially shaped wires in their underwire bras for additional support. These companies have conducted market research and found that an oval wire provides better support in the larger sizes. Whenever you're shopping, examining how a bra is constructed can help to measure its quality.

Fabric

Like with any piece of clothing, the cost of the fabric has a variable affect on the cost of your bra. Inexpensive cotton will cost less than a filmy silk. But there are other aspects to consider. Cotton is easier to work with, making the workmanship less expensive than with silk. The fabric is also a key indicator of quality because what you're actually looking for is a fabric that doesn't stretch too much. Higher end brands will often add a layer of mesh or other supportive fabric into the band of larger cup-size bras to improve the garment's support. Those additions add to the quality and cost.

According to Claire Terentiev, Head of Design at Chantelle, "When developing a new bra, we think about the larger sizes when we choose the fabrics, straps, details, etc. What is equally important is that the aesthetics of the bra remain the same from small to large sizes. The width of the straps and backs evolve as the size gets larger, but we never compromise the aesthetic of the bra. We add linings and other reinforced materials inside the bra, which adds cost and complication for our production teams, but it makes for a superior product."

Embellishments

All of the buttons, bows, and added decorative details on a bra are considered embellishments. Although embellishments may not affect how a bra fits, they do add to the cost of a bra and are pored over as a design choice. Similarly, the lace used in a bra has a direct affect on the cost. Lace can be quite expensive, and the challenging demands of working with such a delicate material are reflected in the final cost of a single lace bra.

Hand Sewing

Some of the specialized tailoring you will find is done by hand, another of the quality factors determining price. The more time each bra takes to construct, and the more expert labor that's needed to sew it, the more expensive it will be. When you're shopping, observe the strength of the stitching and the finesse of the hand sewing as an indicator of quality and durability.

How to Customize Your Fit

Not every bra is going to fit perfectly and that's where a customer-friendly boutique or a great seamstress can play an important role. Some high-end boutiques will make adjustments (sometimes free-of-charge!) with the bras you purchase in their stores. They can shorten or lengthen straps, add pads against the underwire if that's chafing,

For a list of specialized boutiques around the country, go to www.fabfoundations.com/bustedextras

cut down (or even remove) underwires that poke armpits, make band adjustments, or any number of things you may need to ensure a safe and comfortably fitting bra. If you're able to shop in a high-end boutique, don't be shy! Take advantage of their services.

The Most Economical Piece in Your Wardrobe

Instead of focusing on which bra will provide the best fit, Americans tend to go for quantity, trying to capitalize on "Buy One, Get One Free" offers and other promotions.

While many women may balk at the idea of spending a lot of money on a bra, if you break it down to its cost-per-wear, bras are probably one of the most economical pieces in your wardrobe.

The price of bras range across a wide spectrum, from less than $20 to well over $200, and you can find quality garments at an array of prices.

Let's assume you purchase a good-quality $70 bra. At $70, that's a pricey garment, but don't focus on that for now. Just think about the cost from this perspective: if cared for properly, that bra will last for approximately 150 to 200 wearings. That works out to less than 40 cents per wearing—40 cents for a garment that will improve your looks and your health. When you compare that cost to other daily expenses, say, a cup of coffee, then purchasing a higher quality bra seems much more affordable, doesn't it?

Conversely, a cheaply constructed bra, no matter how well you take care of it, will not provide excellent support for anywhere near as long. If only life was simple enough that the price tag on a bra was a true indicator of its quality. Sadly, that's not the case. There are pricey bras of lesser quality and bargains that are well constructed. It can be confusing. In the long run, a lesser quality garment will lose its elasticity more quickly, and the fabric may stretch out or fade, making its cost-per-wear much higher. Part of The FabFit™ Formula is understanding quality markers, as outlined above, which will guide you to high-quality bras at any price point.

Ask Ali

Q: I went to a lingerie store and it seemed like all the bras cost at least $100! My eyes bugged out of my head!!
When you talk about buying a quality bra, does that mean I have to spend that kind of cash?

Thanks for your help,
Liana, San Mateo, CA

A: Quality and cost do not always go hand in hand. Oftentimes, expensive bras are worth every penny. However, there are inexpensive bras of wonderful quality, and extremely costly bras that may be gorgeous but are designed more for fashion than fit. Always try on a bra to assess fit and demand quality merchandise—at a price point that is comfortable for you.

How Much Should You Spend on a Bra?

When it comes to buying bras, it helps to do some research. Ask your friends where they shop. Generally speaking, you should think about your budget.

So what does that mean for you? First, commit to buying a bra that fits. When you focus on the fit factors, you will improve how you look in feel. And that's true at any price. Once you see the difference that fit makes, you may be tempted to upgrade the quality of your garment, because higher quality bras will keep you lifted longer and that provides better value.

"Buy the best quality bra you can afford," says Sarah Weiner of Trousseau, "because a higher quality bra will maintain its structure and save you money long term."

When you see how you look in your garments and become willing to invest in better fit, it's a way of showing that you value yourself.

Most women don't just go shopping; they walk into the dressing room with a lot of preconceived notions about their bodies and their self-image. Bra shopping is no exception. If anything, it magnifies how we view ourselves, because bras speak to our core ideas about being a woman and how we measure up—or don't.

"Shopping is an emotional process as well as behavioral, and it's complicated," says Ellen Jacobson of Elila. "If bra shopping was easy, then the numbers of women buying the wrong size wouldn't be so high."

It's All About the Fit

Because bra shopping can be such an emotional experience, women sometimes resist looking honestly at their bodies. Some might focus on what size they wish to be instead of considering their actual best fit. Others obsess over every bulge and have unrealistic expectations. Then they blame the bra when the fit isn't right.

Not every person can wear every bra, even if it's the right size. The cut of the bra and your own body play major roles in the final equation.

The way to keep this from being confusing is to focus on the fit of the bra, not the size. It's all about the fit.

Be flexible about your bra size, as all brands (and styles) fit differently. Try not to walk into a store with too many preconceived ideas. This should be a pleasurable experience and not something to be dreaded, like going to the dentist. Be prepared to be surprised and have fun!

—Frederika Zappé, National Fit Specialist, Eveden, Inc.

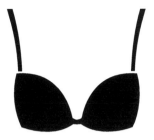

7

Essential Steps to Stress-Free Bra Shopping

*N*ow that you know what you're looking for, it's time to put your FabFit™ Formula to work and go shopping! For your first outing, put those two-for-one deals away (for now) and find the store nearest you with the widest range of bra brands. Ideally, look for an establishment that puts an emphasis on bra fit, like an upscale lingerie boutique or one of the better department stores.

The FabFit™ Formula in Action

1. Find a store that carries a wide variety of brands in a range of price points.

2. Nothing replaces a professional fitter with a good eye and abundant knowledge about merchandise, but there's no way to know if your fitter is any good until you're in the dressing room and give her a legitimate chance. If your fitter is less than optimal, which can happen even in a store with a great reputation, remember The FabFit™ Formula. That way, you'll take care of yourself, and that's very empowering.

3. A great fitter (or even one who is not so hot) can bring you sizes that will fit your body, no matter what the national origin of the bra. She should also be able to tell you what styles might look best on your shape, and which brands cater best to your body and breast type.

4. The first time you go shopping using The FabFit™ Formula, assume you don't know which bras will fit you best. Be open-minded and try a wide array of styles and sizes, even if they are very different from the ones you usually wear.

For more information about stores near you, go to
www.fabfoundations.com/bustedextras

Fitting the Band

As you begin to try on bras, think about your band size. Since you know what size you've been wearing, you have a starting point with the bras you already own.

* Is the band on your current bra firm, anchored, and horizontal?

* Is it loose or tight?

Based on your answers, find some bras with band sizes that correspond to what you think your band size might be. For now, you're ignoring the cup size. Just focus on the band. Take several bras, including a couple of your best guesses for band size, into the dressing room. You're going to try on the bra backward. This will help you isolate the fit of the band while ignoring the cups. Don't put the straps on your shoulders; make sure the band is sitting directly under your breasts, where it would normally be. If you try the band on below the point where it should be sitting, you'll never get your best fit: firm, anchored, and horizontal.

* Focusing on the band only, assess the feel.

* Is it secure without being uncomfortably tight?

* Do you get immediate resistance when you pull the band away from your body?

* Can you pull it away from your body by more than an inch or two?

When shopping for a new a bra, the row of hooks you use when fastening the band makes a big difference in the overall fit. Many women think that they should try on bras using the tightest hook. In fact, the opposite is true. You want to buy a bra using the loosest hook that fits your body. The reason is that a bra stretches as it ages, and a bra can be tightened as it stretches, insuring a longer life span. Ideally, a new bra will fit you best on the loosest hook, giving the fabric the most opportunity for give. Women's bodies, however, come in too many shapes and sizes to make this a universal rule.

Try a variety of band sizes until you find the one that seems to feel consistently firm, anchored, and horizontal on your rib cage. You will not always wear this band size (because the focus is on fit), so once you find a bra with a band that does fit you can move on to fitting your cups, bridge, and straps.

You may find that the store where you're shopping doesn't carry bras that correspond to your rib-cage size. If that's the case, find the closest possible band size the store offers and pull the bra around your body, with the cups in the back. If you need a larger size, measure the amount of space that is left exposed between the two ends of the band. Add the number of inches left uncovered to the size of that bra band to estimate your band size. Since bands are measured in even numbers, if the amount of exposed skin is an odd number of inches, you'll want to start by looking at bras that round up to the next even number. For example, if you tried on a bra with a 40-band, and you had approximately three inches of skin left uncovered, begin by looking at bras with a 44-band.

If the smallest band is too big, measure the amount that the band overlaps across your body. Subtract those inches of overlap from the band size. That difference is the band size you should try to find. If the amount of overlap is an odd number then round to the next larger number. In other words, if you tried on a 32-band bra and there were three inches of overlap, start with a 30-band bra.

These are starting points, and trying on the bra itself is the only way to check for fit.

Finding Your Cup Size

Now that you have figured out your band size, it's time to focus on the cup. Look again at the bra you had when you started shopping. The cup size and the band size are interrelated, so the cup on a 36B is the same as a 34C and a 32D. For each band size you may have moved up or down in the previous exercise, adjust your cup size accordingly to get back to the same cup size as your existing bra. If you were wearing a 36C and now find yourself in a 34-band, then a D-cup will have the same cup size as your existing bra. Conversely, if you were wearing a 32B and found that you went up a band size, you should now be wearing a 34A.

If you already knew your cup size was too small or too large based on The FabFit™ Formula, then adjust your size by trying bras that are larger or smaller in the cup, according to what you think you need. Test the cup fit by pressing along the line of the underwire or the outline of the cup on a soft bra. This will ensure that the bra is capturing all of your breast tissue.

Once you have a band/cup combination that seems like a winner, test whether the band is carrying the recommended 80 to 90 percent of the weight of your breasts. Then slip your straps off your shoulders. Although your breasts may move, the band should stay in its firm, anchored, and horizontal position. If the band slips, it's an indication that the fit is not yet Fab.

You may need to try on a large number of bras—in a variety of sizes—before finding your best fit. This process can be time consuming, especially for your first shopping expedition, but knowing that you thoroughly understand how to fit yourself can help reduce—and even eliminate—the stress involved in bra shopping. The FabFit™ experience will give you the confidence that you can find the right fit for your body. When you become more familiar with your unique shape, and with the brands and sizes that work best for you, shopping will become more efficient.

Jennifer Learns a Lesson

Remember Jennifer, the high school basketball player you read about in chapter 2?

After some frustrating shopping experiences, she decided to use what she had learned from The FabFit™ Formula. She found a store that claimed to be all about fit. Upon arrival, the fitter brought Jennifer into the dressing room, took her measurements, and announced her bra size. As Jenny began trying on bras, she quickly realized that they didn't fit correctly. The cups were too small, the middle didn't lie flat against her body, and the band was loose. At first, she felt frustrated. After the saleswoman insisted that she knew the correct size, Jenny began fighting back tears. Then she realized that she had learned a formula for success that she could put to use. Jenny was able to find some great bras that fit, and she left the store feeling comfortable, confident, and empowered.

The Fab Fit™ Assessment

When your cup and band combination seems to fit, ask these key questions:

- Is the band firm, anchored, and horizontal?
- Is the band doing 80 to 90 percent of the work to support your breasts?
- If you are wearing an underwire bra, does the bridge lay flat against your breastbone?
- Have you placed all of your breast tissue in the cup by gently lifting your breasts and dropping them into the cup?
- Are the cups doing their job to capture everything?
- Are your straps adjusted to be firm but not tight? (No more than 10 to 20 percent of the support?)

You should be answering YES to the questions above.

Now move around in the bra, as you would normally, over the course of a day.

- Is the bra uncomfortable?
- Does anything dig in?
- Does the band rise up?
- Does the cup cut into your tissue or does your breast slip out in any way?

You should be answering NO to the questions above.

Otherwise, you should keep looking for another bra or another size.

Is It the Right Bra for You?

Once you can answer yes to the first set of questions and
no to the second, you probably have the right size bra for
your body in that particular style. But is it the right bra
for you? Look at the bra itself. Are the back wings cutting into the flesh on your back? If so, you may not have a
wide enough back band. If it feels like the band is taking
over your back unnecessarily—and ultimately the width
of your band is a judgment call—then perhaps the band is
too wide. This is not a matter of weight; this is just how
your body is proportioned.

Is the cup style providing a pleasing shape for your
taste and the contours of your body? If you need the bra
to perform a particular task—i.e., smooth cup or plunge—
will it do the trick?

If you are wearing an underwire bra, does the entire
bridge tack to your body, or does it gap anywhere? If
it gaps, you might need to experiment with bras featuring wider or narrower bridges. Soft cup wearers, does
your bridge stay close to your body, without being visible
beneath your clothing or creating a third "cup" between
your breasts?

Once you have a bra that seems like a contender, try it
on with a plain T-shirt or with an outfit that you may be
purchasing to go with it. A bra needs to look great under
your preferred set of clothes.

There is a key exception to this rule. Sometimes,
women choose lingerie expressly for its singular effect when
not being worn with clothes. If your bra is for purposes
independent of your wardrobe, just be clear on what job

you need that bra to do and make a selection that will best suit its purpose.

Once all of the other FabFit™ factors are in place, ask yourself what many women consider to be the most important question: Is this bra comfortable?

You should never buy an uncomfortable bra. You may need to get used to wearing a firm band, and a band may leave marks on your skin for a short time after removing it, but a properly fitted bra should feel comfortable. If it doesn't feel right in the store, imagine how miserable you'll be after wearing it for hours on end. It's just like buying shoes a size too small. You might convince yourself in the store that they'll work just fine, but before long, you'll be sorry and most likely in pain.

Once you've purchased the bra that's right for you, it's vital to know exactly how to wear it. It may seem counterintuitive to discuss something that sounds so basic, especially since most of you have been wearing a bra for a long time. But please read on. You may find a few surprises.

How to Put On Your Bra

1. Start by placing the straps loosely on your shoulders.
2. Bend at the waist and let your breasts fall into the cups.
3. As you stand, fasten the bra behind your back.
4. Use your left hand to reach into the far side of your right cup. Lightly pull your breast tissue up and gently drop it, letting the tissue settle naturally into the cup. You want to make sure that you're pulling all of the excess breast tissue from underneath your

armpit. But be kind to your girls! You don't want to pull roughly at your delicate breast tissue. Now repeat on the other side.

5.   Smooth down the cleavage area to make sure that there are no lumps and bumps.

6.   Look in the mirror to ensure that your nipples are set in the middle of the cup, pointing straight out, at a 90-degree angle from your body.

7.   Adjust your straps to be firm but not tight. You should get into the habit of adjusting your straps every time you put on your bra, as the strap rings can loosen with wear and washing.

8.   Voila!

If you put your bra on by hooking it in the front and twisting the hooks to the back, you can damage your bra. It's better if you can hook it in the back because the twisting action stretches the band out faster. A lot of women hop out of the shower and attempt to put on their bra while they're still wet, so their bra sticks on their damp body. It's not fun to wrestle with a bra first thing in the morning and it's not great for the bra, either.

Frederika Zappé, National Fit Specialist for the Eveden brands, suggests a great trick: if you're unable to hook your bra behind your back—and many women can't—try hooking the bra in front over either a slip or panty hose or something that will facilitate you shifting the position of the band so that you can rotate the bra without stretching it.

Making Internet Shopping Work for You

Many women may not find the size or style they need in a local store. Others may want a wider selection. Internet shopping is the way to address either of those issues.

Here are ten tips to help you figure out what to order when shopping online.

1. Go to any local store and use the method described to estimate your band size.
2. Oftentimes, the key to finding the best size for you to purchase is to start with the bras you already own. If you're currently wearing a 36C, and you've realized that you should really be in a 32-band, then you'll be going down two band sizes. Compensate for the changed band size by trying bras that are two cup sizes larger—a DD or E— depending upon the brand (see chart on pages 106-107). In any case, you now have a target band size and a target cup size.
3. For some women, particularly those with cup sizes larger than a D-cup, this method doesn't work, and some may feel as if they will never find a bra that fits. Ideally, you should try to find a store with a wide range of bra sizes to determine your approximate size. If online shopping is your only option, then try this: Put on your best, unpadded, non-contour bra. Take a tape measure and measure across the fullest part of your breast, over your nipple. The tape measure must be parallel to the ground all the way around your body, so you might want to enlist a friend to help, or do it in front of a mirror. You want the measuring tape to be just firm enough around your body that

it won't slip off, but no tighter. The tape should not press into your skin.

4. Subtract the number of your bust measurement from your band size. The difference between your band size and this new measurement represents one cup size per inch.

5. **This is NOT your size, this is your starting point.** It's important—no, it's imperative—to remember that measurement is no substitute for fit, particularly for a full-breasted woman. This is just one step in the process.

6. Go online to a website with a wide range of options, while taking note of its current return policy. The website www.fabfoundations.com has links to a number of sites with an excellent selection of merchandise.

7. Find a few bras in various styles, using the tips in chapter 5 to identify shapes that might work better for your body.

8. Order the bras in several sizes that are close to the starting size you identified. You may end up ordering a large number of bras, but you'll be returning most of them, so be particular about handling the bras with care once they arrive.

To download your own printable copies of the charts from this chapter, go to www.fabfoundations.com/bustedextras

9. When your bras arrive, start by fitting the band and only then assess the cups, bridge, and straps.

10. Try on the variety of sizes and styles with a critical eye, using The FabFit™ Formula.

Cup Size Measurement Chart	
The difference between your band size and this new measurement represents one cup size per inch.	
Less than ½"	AAA cup
½-1"	AA cup
1"	A cup
2"	B cup
3"	C cup
4"	D cup

Which Cup Size Should I Buy?

If your cup size is larger than a D-cup, then you'll find that cup size progression differs between brands. The chart on pages 106-107 will help you determine which sizes are equivalent and will also give you a sense of which manufacturers produce bras in your size.

Similarly for petite-bra wearers, size is often inconsistent from brand to brand. Check out page 105 for a comparison of how the major petite-bra manufacturers tend to fit.

Considering Your Cycle

Your body changes over the course of its monthly cycle. If you are someone who swells significantly when menstruating, you should take that into account when timing your shopping. You may also opt to try bras with more stretch in the cups, knowing that you're going to expand

and contract over the course of each month. Some women increase in size by one or two cups with each cycle. If that's you, consider buying a dedicated bra for that time of the month. Either way, remember your monthly cycle when you go shopping for a bra.

Ask Ali

Q: You say that The FabFit™ Filosofy means no measuring, but then you tell women to measure to find their cup size. What's up with that?

Carolyne
Chicago, IL

A: Great question! There's a fundamental difference between standard bra size calculators, which use a measurement to establish cup size, and The FabFit™ Formula. In the formula, the measurement is only one step in the process of deciding which bras to purchase for trial; it's not a determination of your definitive size. Until you've tried a bra on your body and have a sense of what size tends to fit you, bra shopping online is hard! Understand that the cup measurement is just one step in the fit process. Ultimately, taking a measurement and thinking you have FabFit™ is like running a race and stopping before the finish line.

Trial and Error

It is difficult to order bras online while you are still determining your best fit. The first time may be time consuming and may not yield your ultimate fit.

While FabFitT is a tried and true formula; it is subject to the unique qualities of each individual. There is always a certain amount of trial and error, particularly in the beginning. That's why it's so helpful to experiment in a boutique that stocks an array of bras in your size range.

As Franchesca Carrasquillo, of The Full Cup in Virginia Beach, Virginia, says, "Unless you try, you'll never know, so keep trying new things.

PETITE BRA CUP-SIZE COMPARISON, BY BRAND

If your cup size is a... ...then buy a	AAA	AA	A	B	C
Itty Bitty Bra*	AA	A	B		
Lula Lu Petites	AAA	AA	A	B	C
Mimi Holliday by Damaris		A	B	C	
The Little Bra Company**		A	B	C	
Timpa Duet		A	B	C	
Wacoal Petites***		AA	A	B	C

* Tends to run small in the cup
** Tends to run small in the band
*** Tends to run larger than other petite bras

Courtesy: Amanda Sage Barnum, 32aabra.com.

Difference Between Bust and Band

Manufacturer	4"	5"	6"	7"	8"	9"	10"	11"	12"	13"	14"
Alegro	D	DD	E	F	FF	G	GG	H			
Anita	D	E	F	G	H						
Aviana	D	DD/E	DDD/F	G	H	I	J	K	L		
Bali	D	DD	DDD								
Bendon Sport	D	DD	E	F	FF	G					
Chantelle	D	E	F	G	H						
Conturelle	D	E	F	G	H	I					
Curvation	D	DD	DDD								
Elila	D	E	F	G	H	I	J	K	L	M	N
Elle MacPherson	D	DD	E	F	FF	G					
Elomi	D	DD	E	F	FF	G	GG	H	HH	J	JJ
Empreinte	D	E	F	G							
Exquisite Form	D	DD	DDD								
Fancee Free	D	DD/E	DDD/F	G	H	I	J	K	L		
Fantasie	D	DD	E	F	FF	G	GG	H	HH	J	JJ
Fauve	D	DD	E	F	FF	G	GG	H	HH	J	JJ
Fayreform	D	DD	E	F	FF	G	GG	H	HH	J	
Felina	D	DD	DDD								
Freya	D	DD	E	F	FF	G	GG	H	HH	I	JJ

Chart Courtesy of BiggerBras.com.

Difference Between Bust and Band

Manufacturer	4"	5"	6"	7"	8"	9"	10"	11"	12"	13"	14"
Goddess	D	DD	DDD	G	H	I	J	K	L	M	N
Grenier	D	DD/E	DDD/F								
Harlequin	D	DD	E	F	FF	G	GG	H	HH	J	JJ
Kris	D	DD	E	F	FF	G	GG	H	HH	J	JJ
Le Mystere	E	E	F	G	H						
Leading Lady	D	DD/E	DDD/F	G	H	I					
Marie Jo	D	E	F	G							
Mia	D	DD	DDD	G	H						
Natori	D	DD	DDD	G							
Panache	D	DD	E	F	FF	G	GG	H	HH	J	JJ
Playtex	D	DD	DDD								
Prima Donna	D	E	F	G	H	I					
Royce Bras	D	DD	E	F	FF	G	GG	H	HH	J	JJ
Shock Absorber	D	DD	E	F	FF	G	GG	H	HH		
Simone Perele	D	E	F								
Va Bien	D	DD	DDD								
Vanity Fair	D	DD	DDD								
Venus	D	DD/E	DDD/F								
Wacoal	D	DD	E	F	G	H	I				

For an expanded, printable chart, please visit www.fabfoundations.com/bustedextras

Chart Courtesy of BiggerBras.com. The chart lists common cup sizes as measured BiggerBras.com and should be used as a guide only.

It's all about a good foundation, whether it's a body or a house. My job as a designer is to make a woman feel her best because if she's not comfortable, it will shine through. Ultimately, if you're fussing, you're not at your best.

—Scott Overgaard,
Hollywood Stylist and Image Consultant

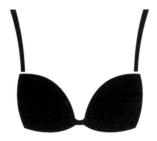

8

How To Save Your Bra from an Untimely Death

The lifespan of your bra depends upon three things: the quality of its manufacturing, your rate of wear and tear, and your laundry habits. This chapter will explain how to take care of your garment, insuring maximum support, value, and staying power.

Give Your Bra a Break

If you want your bra to last, keep it cool. Heat is an elastic-killer and the number-one cause of bra death. Think about it. Your bra sits on your body for many hours at a time, stuck somewhere in the 95 to 100 degree range—no matter what the weather may be. This amount of heat can wear out a bra when it's worn for several days in a row.

So how about giving your bra a break on a regular basis? Wear a bra one day; then let it sit for at least 24 hours. Resting your bra will preserve its elastic and help you retain the firm support you need.

Washing Tips

You should wash a bra after every other wearing. Some women tend to over do it, washing a bra after every wear. Over-washing will shorten the life of many delicate garments, including your bras. If you've sweated—or as some might say, "glowed" — then, yes, please, wash your bra. Otherwise, the industry recommendation is to wash your bra after every other wearing.

How—exactly—do you wash your bra?

In an ideal world, you would hand wash it in cool water, using a specially formulated lingerie wash, then line dry it over molds that retain the shape of your cups.

Lingerie wash is unique compared to delicate washing formulas designed for other fabrics, such as wool. The properties needed to hand wash wool differ from what's needed for elastic and other delicate materials like silk or lace. There are a number of lingerie washes out there, including Forever New and Le Blanc, that can usually be found in lingerie boutiques, better department stores, and online. Some stores have in-house brands, and there are other excellent products on the market. What they all have in common is that they are formulated expressly for lingerie.

Many women simply can't be bothered to hand wash their delicates. The next best alternative to hand washing, which is a perfectly acceptable way to go, is to launder bras in a lingerie bag on the delicate cycle, if your washing machine has one. If it doesn't, use cold water and the gentlest possible cycle. There are some nice, big lingerie bags out there in consumer land, so you can launder a number of your delicates together.

Whenever you use a lingerie bag, don't stuff it. Leave plenty of room for your delicates to move around, so the water and cleaning agent can move freely through the garments. That's what gets them clean.

Follow two more golden rules to preserve the life of your favorite purchases.

* Never use bleach. It breaks down the fibers and the elastic.

* Always close the hooks of your bras when you wash them. Not only will that maintain the shape; it will also prevent your bra hooks from snagging on other garments.

Let's face it: when life gets in the way, hand washing with special lingerie wash doesn't always happen. You may not have time to do any laundry at all. If that's the case, try this alternative. Wear your bra into the shower and use baby shampoo (or even soap) on the bra while you shower. Rinse and air-dry. This shortcut is particularly useful on the road.

Dryers and Delicates: A Lethal Combination

Air-dry your bras. Always. Putting lingerie of any kind in a hot dryer is like sentencing it to death. It is also recommended that you do not dry clean or iron your bra because heat will damage its elasticity and wreck its shape, particularly a bra with a formed cup.

After washing, pat your delicates dry, but don't wring them out or twist them. You can damage the fragile fabric, not to mention the havoc you will wreak on the structure of a bra. Twisted underwires are not comfortable.

When air-drying, lay your garment flat or hang it up. Laying a contoured-cup bra flat retains the shape of its form.

The violence of the dryer can also weaken the fabric that keeps an underwire securely in place, allowing it to break free, causing a most unpleasant poking sensation in one of your most delicate body parts. Once an underwire has broken free, the bra is, essentially, destroyed. Any woman who has endured a day of feeling like a pincushion can attest to that unique discomfort.

One last reminder: heat hurts!

For a list of FabFit™ cleaning tips, go to
www.fabfoundations.com/bustedextras

More Tips for a Long-Lasting Bra

Here are some more steps you can take to maintain and extend the usefulness of your bra.

A good seamstress can lengthen the life of a bra by adding an additional row of hooks and eyes to keep your band secure even after it stretches. Adjustable rings on straps can also be replaced, if needed.

When you take good care of your lingerie, it extends its life and the financial value you receive from your purchase. That's true at any price point. If your bra lasts longer, it needs to be replaced less often and that saves you money. Of course, if you're buying low-cost, low-quality bras, proper care will certainly help, but your bras will wear out faster and need to be replaced more often than a better quality garment. At a certain point, you'd be better off simply buying a better quality bra that will last longer. If a higher quality bra will also provide better support, then multiple factors might point toward seeing a bra as an investment in yourself and your wardrobe.

As previously discussed, a bra lasts for approximately six months of wearings. Let's say that equals thirty days per month times six months. In other words, 180 wearings. A seventy-dollar bra worn 180 times costs approximately 39 cents per wearing. If you wear that bra every other day, your quality bra costs less than six dollars each month. Those six dollars will not only make you look and feel better every day; in the long run, it will improve your physical and emotional health.

This is not to suggest that you must spend seventy dollars as the magic price for a quality bra. There are many great bras on the market that cost more or less than seventy dollars. By using that price as an example, your cost per wear makes a quality bra a better buy. After all, how much do you spend on coffee or snacks each month?

When to Replace Your Bra

Most American women don't take proper care of their bras and wait too long before replacing them. FabFit™ is not just about helping you find a bra that gives you the support and shape you need; it's about keeping it in great condition and making it last.

So when should you replace a bra? That depends upon the quality of the garment and how you care for it. A bra should last for at least six months of normal wear and tear. If you wear a bra every other day, it should last approximately one year. Oftentimes, a quality garment that is well cared for will last longer than that. But instead of checking your calendar to determine when you should replace a garment, examine it carefully for the necessary clues. Replace your bra whenever you notice any of the following:

- When the elastic in your bra is going or gone. You'll know that's happening when you see little white threads of elastic showing through the fabric. If you get to the point where the elastic makes a crunching sound when it stretches, you've waited far too long.

- If the fabric of the bra is stretched out and doesn't bounce back after wearing it, or when you test the fabric by pulling on it. If there's no give in the band, it can't move with you and provide the support you need.

- If your band is still loose at its tightest hook, either replace the bra or try to extend its life through alterations. Once the band can no longer provide a firm, anchored, and horizontal fit, it's time for it to go.

- When the underwire is misshapen or poking out, it's all over. Once an underwire has broken free, your bra is a goner. Yes, you can attempt to stitch it back in, and maybe you can wring a few more wearings out of it, but it's more or less toast.

- If your bra is discolored or faded, it's probably worn out.

- Don't keep an uncomfortable bra, even if it was expensive. Even if you got it for your bridal shower or you saw it written up in a fashion magazine, if a bra feels uncomfortable, so will you, and you won't be at your best. People may not know your bra is the problem; they will just know that you are somehow off your game. When is a good time for that?

- If your bra doesn't fit, replace it. Period. Women have a tendency to hang on to clothes that don't fit, promising themselves that "One day, I'll fit into these jeans again." When it comes to your bra, there's no rule that says you can't keep it, but after a few years, regardless of whether or not you wear it, time takes its toll on the elastic in a bra. The garment simply can't do its job effectively when the elastic no longer provides support.

No two boobs are alike, even on the same body.

—Elisabeth Dale, author of bOObs:
A Guide to Your Girls, and founder of TheBreastLife.com

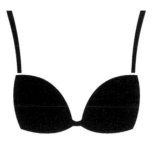

9

Bras Through a Lifetime: Revisiting The FabFit™ Filosofy

As a woman's body changes, she may need to adjust her choice of bras, and unforeseen lifestyle issues may require a specialty bra. The FabFit™ Formula can help with any of these unique challenges.

Your First Bra

Asking a woman about her experience shopping for her first bra can unleash a torrent of horror stories. Positive recollections are few and far between, and that's a shame because those initial shopping outings can impact a girl's self-esteem for many years.

Back when the average age for girls getting their periods was older than it is now, it made sense for parents and educators to introduce talk of the birds and the bees with the onset of the monthly cycle. Nowadays, as girls hit puberty from age eight and up, the conversation must change. Some mothers still choose to initiate talk about sex while taking their daughters on those first shopping trips for a bra. But such focused scrutiny can make a youngster feel extremely self-conscious. If you're talking to an elementary school child about her new bra, she's probably not thinking about becoming a young woman; she's much more inclined to be concentrating on recess and what's on television.

Because most girls are shopping for bras long before they are ready to be sexually active, the potential for mixed messages is rather high. Eventually, a girl will discover that how she feels about her breasts is an integral part of how she feels about herself as a woman. That's why bra shopping at such an early age can become so loaded.

The Teen Years and Training Bras

The puberty shift to younger ages has also affected the marketing of training bras. Until the 1960s, manufacturers focused on 13- to 19-year-olds as first-time bra purchasers. Within two decades, the targeted age range had been lowered to 10- to 13-year olds. Now, even younger girls have a need for bras, introducing emotional turmoil to a new group of younger and younger girls.

In order to make that first shopping trip a pleasant experience, the adult must send a positive message that wearing a bra is all about health and feeling good about oneself.

Here are three tips to help make that first outing a success:

1. Pick a store that carries merchandise in sizes that work for your daughter. Some stores stock first-bra styles, while others stock petite bras that might fit your teen's body, but are not in age appropriate styles or fabrics. A little advance research about a store's inventory will simplify what could become an unnecessarily emotional outing.

2. Find a salesperson who relates to your daughter with minimal embarrassment. Reserving an appointment gives everyone a chance to think about who will be the best assistant for your daughter and which merchandise will suit her needs.

3. As your daughter grows, be prepared if she feels insecure about her figure. Girls are exquisitely sensitive and uncertain about the changes in their bodies, and shopping for bras can provide a great opportunity to enforce positive messages about body image, no matter how much or how quickly a girl's body is developing— or not. In the case of rapid development, new bras may be required.

Weight Gain and Loss

Bodies can change at any age. A weight fluctuation of as little as five pounds can affect a woman's bra size, yet women often resist purchasing new bras when they gain or lose weight. Sometimes, it's because they don't understand the importance of FabFit™. Others may not want to spend money unnecessarily. All too often, the reason women choose not to replenish their bra wardrobe has to do more with feeling like they haven't yet earned the right.

If you are gaining or losing weight, having a properly fitting bra will provide you with comfort and support, which will, in turn, make you look and feel more confident. No matter what the reason for your weight change, acquiring external support will insure a better chance of increased emotional health.

Sports Bras

Weight loss can sometimes be related to increased fitness, but any time a woman exercises, it is imperative that she wear a properly fitted sports bra.

Have you ever watched a woman jog down the street, breasts bouncing in a way that can only be described as painful? Ouch! Why go through that torture? Particularly when fantastic exercise bras are out there in a range of sizes and styles.

A sports bra is an essential garment for any woman who exercises, but many women never think to buy properly fitted bras for their workouts. In fact, research has revealed that 73 percent of women who work out regularly do not wear sports bras. According to Sarah Weiner from Trousseau, "Some women wear old bras as sports bras, but that's the worst thing you can do." Old bras are already stretched beyond their ability to provide adequate support, so they certainly won't hold up to the job of giving you the support you need during an active workout.

A sports bra significantly reduces breast movement and accompanying pain when exercising. Repetitive motion can also increase the rate of damage to delicate breast tissue, causing sagging and stretch marks. Even an A-cup woman can get vertical stretch marks if she doesn't take care of her breasts.

More than half of women joggers report breast pain. Some women choose not to exercise because of the discomfort it brings. This doesn't have to happen! A properly fitting sports bra can significantly reduce breast movement and any associated pain, making exercise more comfortable and healthy. These days, women can find great sports bras in a wide variety of sizes, from an A-cup to a K-cup. *The Journal of Science and Medicine in Sports* has done extensive research on this subject and their findings strongly support the use of sports bras for active women.

There are two main kinds of sports bras: compression and encapsulation. Compression bras do exactly what their name implies; they compress the tissue tightly against the body, making it more difficult for the breasts to move. Compression bras aren't ideal for well-endowed women. Anyone larger than a C-cup should strongly consider an encapsulation style bra. They are built and sized more like a standard bra, with each breast encased in an individual cup. Encapsulation bras feature bands with hooks and eyes and adjustable straps.

Ask Ali

Q: How do I know when it's time to replace a sports bra?

Marla

Frederick, MD

A: Sports bras exist to do the job of holding your breasts firmly in place while you exercise. They perform an important job so replacing them at the right time is critical to your breast health. The job of the sports bra is a balance between providing enough stretch as your body moves and adequate tension to offer proper support. As your sports bra ages, you will eventually end up with a stretched out bra that has lost its elasticity and support. If that's the case, the time has come to replace your sports bra.

Hormonal Changes

As discussed in chapter 7, every woman has a unique reaction to her monthly cycle and changes in her breasts. For some, a bra with a more flexible cup is enough. Others may need a dedicated bra in a different cup size to get them through. Ultimately, it's knowing your own body and how your bras fit throughout the month that determine your best course of action.

In addition to normal hormonal fluctuations, going on or off birth control can affect a woman's breast size. If this causes enough change in your size that your bras no longer work, go back to your FabFit™ Formula to ensure that you have bras are that are supportive and comfortable.

Maternity and Nursing Bras

When it comes to bras, pregnancy creates changes like nothing else. Bra fit under normal circumstances is hard enough, but the protocol for fitting a constantly growing body is particularly challenging.

Maternity bras are often confused with nursing bras, but they are very different. Maternity bras are specifically designed to accommodate the body's growth during pregnancy, and nursing bras have special clips that offer a baby access to the breast while also providing modesty and minimal fuss for the mother.

Manufacturers recommend that women switch to maternity bras in the third or fourth month of pregnancy. It's a personal choice, dictated by comfort and the extent to which your body is changing. Averages mean little when you're talking about your own body's response to pregnancy, but it's fair to say that pregnant women should expect their bra size to increase in both band and cup size.

A good rule of thumb is to purchase a maternity bra when pre-pregnancy garments become uncomfortable. Unlike the fit procedure for most bras, maternity bras should be tried on the tightest hook, in order to loosen the bra as the ribcage swells to accommodate the growing baby.

For your own convenience, nursing bras should be purchased in advance of your baby's birth, since most women have little interest in shopping once they get home from the hospital. During your first six to eight weeks of nursing, you should expect your cup size to increase an additional one to two sizes from the end of your pregnancy. After approximately eight weeks of nursing, your band size will begin to gradually decrease to its pre-pregnancy size, but your cup size will probably remain larger than it had been before your pregnancy. After nursing, it's important to refit yourself, as many women find that their post-nursing body is different—sometimes drastically—from their pre-pregnancy size.

Tips for Trying on Nursing Bras

Take your feeding schedule into consideration. You want to ensure that your nursing bra will not constrict your breast tissue when you are engorged.

Look for breathable fabrics, such as cotton, to reduce the amount of moisture that builds up in your bra. This will help to prevent infection. Cotton is also recommended to cool the inner fire, as nursing increases the body's temperature.

When shopping, practice using the access clips with one hand, as that will likely be the norm when you're nursing. Quality nursing bras are easily detached and reattached single-handedly.

Find your balance between firm and flexible. On the one hand, a firm fit is critical to comfortably support your larger breasts, but on the other hand, stretch is recommended to accommodate fluctuations in cup size.

Surgical Changes

Anyone who has had her breasts altered by surgery, through augmentation, reduction, or change due to illness, has specific fit issues to consider.

In the year 2010 alone, out of a total of 1.6 million elective plastic surgeries performed in the United States, 31 percent were breast-related. From implants and lifts, to reductions and implant removals, the number of breast surgeries has increased dramatically during the past decade. Many plastic surgeons approach procedures that alter size by breast volume, not bra size. In other words, doctors may not take your band size into consideration when calculating your eventual bra size. This means they are only looking at one part of the bra fit equation, since (as you now know) band and cup size are interrelated. The result is that a woman with a smaller rib cage can ask for one additional cup size, but she may end up a size larger than intended. Conversely, a woman with a larger rib cage may end up with a cup size smaller than what she originally desired.

Directly following your surgery, whether your size is going up or down, it's important to follow your doctor's instructions to ensure speedy recovery. Soft-cup bras made from natural fibers are often recommended during the healing process to prevent pressure and infection.

Once you're cleared by your doctor and back in shopping mode, women with implants might want to purchase bras with materials that breathe more, since implants can be warm. Spacer cups are great options for the augmented set, as they breathe more and form a less rigid shape in the cup.

Prosthesis

If you wear a breast form as a result of a mastectomy or lumpectomy, you can find special bras designed for your needs. Mastectomy bras contain hidden pockets that can house prostheses in one—or both—cups.

But a quality mastectomy bra is more than just a bra with pockets. It is designed with lightweight materials that provide the support and comfort to make your prosthesis look and feel like a natural breast.

After a lumpectomy, many women are confused about how to fit their new shape. Since your breasts may now be different cup sizes, you should fit the larger breast and allow padding or inserts to make up the difference in the smaller breast.

Amoena bras, featuring specially designed "cool fabrics" that equalize body temperature, are ideal for breasts with surgical implants of any kind. Without the ability to respond to temperature changes in the same way as natural breast tissue, the fabric in these bras pulls heat away from a woman's body.

Manufacturers are producing increasingly attractive mastectomy bras, so finding something that feels both comfortable and pretty can help with both the physical and emotional aftermath of surgery.

Sleep Bras

Sleep bras differ from soft-cup bras because they are softer, with less structural support. Experts differ about who (if anyone) should wear a sleep bra. Some say that women should let their breasts "air out" overnight and should never wear sleep bras, while others claim that women, particularly those who are full-busted, need to support their breasts at all times with a bra, even at night. There's also a theory that a woman will damage the delicate ligaments of her breast tissue if she doesn't wear a sleep bra.

According to breast expert Elisabeth Dale, author of bOObs: A Guide to Your Girls and the founder of www. TheBreastLife.com, there is no medical evidence to support the notion that you will damage your breasts without a sleep bra. Dale's position is simple: if you are uncomfortable, you should wear a sleep bra.

Dale and numerous doctors all agree that the decision to wear a sleep bra is a matter of personal preference and comfort, not one based on size.

Ask yourself whether or not you are experiencing breast pain at night. Some women have more pain than others, and occasionally, women go through specific times of increased discomfort, such as in the teen years, when pregnant or nursing, or during menopause. Others experience skin irritation around their breasts during certain times of year. No matter what the cause, identifying tenderness makes the decision to wear a sleep bra much easier. If you are feeling uncomfortable, wear one. Otherwise, there's no need.

Aging

Unfortunately, gravity takes its toll on all of us. As Hollywood image consultant Scott Overgaard says (with his tongue firmly in cheek), "Gravity? It's a drag."

All joking aside; the composition of your breast changes with age. Once a woman's body no longer requires milk production, that dedicated tissue is replaced with fat, which leads to sagging. As your estrogen levels fall, post-menopause, this becomes even more noticeable.

If you've been consistently wearing a properly fitting bra, this is when you will reap the rewards. You'll see fewer changes to your breasts because they will remain lifted longer.

To some extent, the changes that accompany aging are genetic. But whether it's biology or previous habits that have left you hanging lower than you'd like, using The FabFit™ Formula to secure a properly fitting bra will create your best advantage.

*One of the best gifts that a woman can give
to herself is to make sure she's wearing a bra
that fits. Regardless of height, size, or shape,
a properly fitting bra can be life changing in
terms of appearance, comfort, and confidence.*

—Kay-Lin Richardson, Director of Sales, Panache

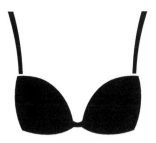

10

The FabFit™ Checklist

*N*ow that you've completed the book, you are ready to assess not only what you have learned but also what you are (hopefully) putting into action. If you can answer YES to everything on this list, you should be feeling great about your bra—and yourself.

The Fab Fit™ Checklist

1. You are focused on how a bra fits you, not the size on the tag.

2. Your band is firm, anchored, and horizontal—and it stays that way.

3. The band is supporting 80 to 90 percent of your bust.

4. Your cups capture all of your breast tissue without any gapping or wrinkles.

5. You put on your bra by scooping all of your breast tissue into the cup.

6. In an underwire bra, the bridge lies flat against your body, even when you raise your hands.

7. Your straps are secure without being tight, carrying only 10 to 20 percent of the weight of your breasts.

8. You readjust your straps every time you put on your bra.

9. Your bra is comfortable when you put it on in the morning and remains that way throughout the day.

10. When shopping, you always try on a bra under your clothes, to see how it fits your body before making the purchase.

11. You think about highlighting your body type with the best bra style for your particular figure.

12. You protect your investment in quality bras by taking good care of them.

Glossary

Guide to Bra Styles

Adhesive or backless bra: A bra without shoulder straps or a rear band, affixed to the breasts with removable adhesive.

Balconette: Also known as a balcony bra, identifiable by wide-set straps and cups that make a straight line across the top of the breasts. Balconettes are great for lifting the bust and are particularly flattering for women with bottom-heavy breasts.

Bandeau: A strapless band of fabric to cover the breasts. Some bandeaus have built-in cups and are most effective for small-busted women.

Bralette: An unlined, soft-cup bra, most often resembling a crop-top. Provides very little support and is generally best for the small-busted. They can also be great sleep bras for women of all sizes.

Contour bra: A bra with a shaped cup that has fiberfill or foam lining. These are highly structured cups that retain the shape of a breast, even when removed from the body. Generally, contour bras have an underwire and can sometimes be known as T-shirt bras. Not to be confused with molded cup bras, contour bras have a sculpted look that can also help reduce "high-beams."

Convertible bra: A bra style featuring removable straps that can be rearranged to fit under a variety of necklines, such as halter-top, one-shoulder, and racer-back. Convertible bras generally double as strapless bras.

Demi-cup bra: "Demi" in French means half and that's exactly what this bra style refers to: a half-cup. These underwire bras expose the top portion of the breast and feature wide-set straps.

Front-clasp/Front-closure bra: Exactly like the name implies, these bras fasten in the front for easier access. Front-clasp bras provide less support than a full cup or seamed bra because they don't offer adjustable band support.

Full cup: A full-cup bra covers most of the breast, providing great support. Full-cup bras were historically recommended for fuller figured women, although that is changing as more manufacturers produce a wider range of styles expressly for full-busted and full-figured women.

Long line: A bra that extends from bust to waist or hips. Generally structured with boning and many hook-and-eye closures. Some long-line bras shape the waist and redistribute the weight of the breasts, making these a great choice for women with back and/or shoulder pain. Bustiers are one type of long-line bra.

Maternity: Designed for pregnant women, these bras feature thicker straps for increased support, which help reduce the breast sensitivity that often comes with pregnancy.

Minimizer: Minimizer bras make the breast appear smaller by pushing breast tissue into a lower-profile cup. Minimizers, in fact, redistribute the breast so that it is spread wider on the chest wall.

Molded: A molded-cup bra is any bra created on a mold. Also referred to as seamless bras or T-shirt bras. Molded-cup bras are often thought of as being interchangeable with contour bras. The difference is that a contour bra is always made with a formed cup that stays in the shape of a breast, even when off the body, while a molded cup can be made from fabric that does not retain its shape. Because they contain no seams, molded-cup bras may not provide as much support for larger-busted women.

Nursing: Designed specifically for women nursing babies. They have some means of supporting the bust while allowing easy access to the nipple for feeding.

Padded: If you want to enhance your shape, push 'em up, or even out asymmetrical breasts, padded bras can do any (or all) of the above by adding fiber, foam, gel, or even air to specific areas of the cup.

Petite bras: In the world of lingerie, petite refers to cup size, rather than height. Petite bras generally provide options for women size B-cup and smaller. Recently, petite manufacturers have begun offering their product in a wider range of band sizes.

Plunge: A bra with a low center, allowing for deeper, v-neck clothes. Plunge bras are also recognizable by their angled cups and narrow center gore/bridge. Unlike padded bras, plunge bras are usually not heavily padded.

Push-up: Just like the name implies, a push-up bra creates lift and cleavage by physically pushing the breasts up and in.

Racer-back: Designed to wear under clothes that reveal shoulder blades and would otherwise expose bra straps.

Seamed/cut and sewn: A bra that is constructed out of pieces that are sewn together to shape and support the breast. Generally speaking, more seams equal more support and more capacity to shape the breast.

Soft cup: Any bra without an underwire, designed to fit all shapes and sizes.

Spacer: A relatively new innovation in the bra market, spacer bras feature two separate fabrics knitted independently, connected by a third, spongy layer. Spacer bras resemble contour bras, but are lighter and breathable. Because the material is breathable, spacer bras provide less nipple coverage than contour bras.

Sports: First introduced in 1977 as a design featuring two jock straps sewn together, sports bras are designed to provide support during physical activity while protecting the breasts from tissue damage. Sports bras come in two designs: compression and encapsulation. Compression bras compress the breasts, pushing them up against the body. Encapsulation looks more like a standard bra, with a distinctive cup for each breast.

Strapless: Designed to be worn without shoulder straps, strapless bras generally have some kind of adhesive agent along the inside edges that adheres the bra to the body.

Terminology

Band: The rear portion of the bra, extending from the cup to the rear hook-and-eye closures. Also known as back wings.

Bridge (aka gore, saddle): The center, front piece of the bra; fabric that connects the cups.

Comfort straps: Bra straps, which are wider than average and can be padded or lined for additional comfort. These are great for full-busted women who are prone to shoulder or neck pain.

Cookies/cutlets: Inserts for bras that can be used to enhance breasts or to even out asymmetrical breasts.

Cups: The area of the bra that holds the breasts.

Extenders: Small rectangles of fabric used to lengthen or reconfigure a back band. Some are used to compensate for an expanding rib cage, while others can convert a standard bra to a low-back bra.

Gore: See bridge.

Petals: Sometimes known as nipple shields. Adhesive-based and stick onto the breast to prevent nipples from showing through clothes. Better than band-aids.

Pole: The place where the strap meets the cup. For example, a center pole is a bra that features straps attached in the center of the cup.

Straps: The part of the bra that extends from the cups, over the shoulders, to the back wings.

Underwire: A thin piece of semi-firm, but flexible, wire that can be fashioned out of any material. The underwire encapsulates the breast and provides support.

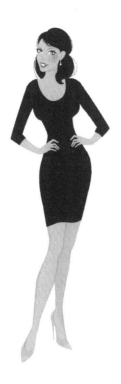

Don't Forget to Visit
www.fabfoundations.com/bustedextras

Resources

Aspan, Rebecca with Sarah Stark. The Lingerie Handbook. Workman Publishing Company, Inc., 2006.

"Bra Fitting? No It Isn't," Which magazine, February, 2010.

Carroll, Jennifer Manuel & Kathy Schultz. Underneath It All: A Girls Guide to Buying, Wearing, And Loving Lingerie. Harlequin Enterprises, Ltd, 2009.

Farrell-Beck, Jane & Colleen Gau. Uplift: The Bra in America. University of Pennsylvania Press, 2002.

Luciani, Jene. The Bra Book: The Fashion Formula to Finding the Perfect Bra. Ben Bella Books, Inc., 2009.

Nethero, Susan. Bra Talk: Myths and Facts: Transform Your Life with the Right Bra Fit. Belle Books, 2005.

Squires, Elisabeth. bOObs: A Guide To Your Girls. Seal Press, 2007.

Holson, Laura M. "Your Bra Size: The Truth May (Pleasantly) Surprise You," The New York Times. April 9, 2009.

Infomat, US Intimates Market Report, 2010.

Infomat. Intimate Apparel: Start a Business.

Monget, Karyn. "Bigger Bras Bolster Sales," Women's Wear Daily. Vol. 199, Issue 61. March 22, 2010.

Medina, Marcy. "Intimacy Plots West Coast Strategy," Women's Wear Daily. April 20, 2009.

Websites

The following websites were used for research and will provide valuable information for those who wish to pursue the subject further.

www.barenecessities.com

The largest online lingerie site, offering a wide selection of lingerie in every available size and price point.

www.amoenamia.com

Amoena's Mia line for information about their innovative cool fabrics.

www.biggerbras.com

A site specializing in the DD+ market.

www.empreinte.eu

Empriente's key points video describes how their products enhance fit.

www.eveden.com

Eveden Brands press release, "British women in need of support"

www.herroom.com

A shopping site offering a wide range of brands and sizes. Owner Tomima Edmark's blog has particularly helpful fit information.

www.lindasonline.com

Linda Becker's shopping site also hosts a superior section for bra-fit problems.

www.wikipedia.com

"Brassiere Measurement" provides a variety of information on the subject, some of which was referenced in Busted!

Acknowledgments

This book couldn't have happened without the love and support of many people.

First and foremost, to my husband, Joe, words will never adequately describe my love, admiration, and respect. The day I sat down next to you in cooking class was the luckiest day of my life.

Mom, thank you for caring so much about everything I say and do. Dad, losing you inspired me to take a leap and write this book. I miss you every day. To my kids, Charleigh and Christian: I love you both so much. Watching you grow up is one of my most profound pleasures. Teddy, you are the best brother a sister could ever ask to have. Joanna, you are my sister in every way, except biological.

To Carol, David, Tess, and Jonathan: thank you for your patience with me as I ditched you to go bra shopping the first time we met, and your careful explanations of which British expressions are family-friendly. I won the in-law family lottery.

To the Kluger boys—Steve, Jeff, Bruce, and Garry—my love and gratitude. Not every girl gets four amazing cousins to coach her through the ups and downs of life. And, Bruce, I will never forget that you were the first to say I was a writer.

Angela Lauria, thank you for your initial excitement about this project, and for staying with me through all its phases. You have been a wonderful friend, sounding board, and publisher.

David Tabatsky, my editor, who reminded me to use my voice. Thanks for ensuring this book's authenticity and overall vision.

To the amazing professionals and colleagues who have been so generous with their time and information:

- Amanda Sage Barnum, 32aabra Blog
- Carla Mackie, The Full Cup, Virginia Beach, VA
- Claire Terentiev, Head of Design, Chantelle Lingerie
- Elisabeth Dale, *bOObs: A Guide to Your Girls*
- Ellen Jacobson, President, Elila
- Ellen Shing, Lula Lu petite lingerie
- Emily Lau, The Little Bra Company
- Francesca Carrasquillo, The Full Cup, Virginia Beach, VA
- Frederika Zappé, National Fit Specialist, Eveden Ltd.
- Kay-Lin Richardson, Director of Sales, Panache
- Layla L'Obatti, Between the Sheets Lingerie
- Sarah Weiner, Trousseau LTD, Vienna, VA
- Scott Overgaard, Stylist and Image Architect
- Treacle, The Lingerie Addict Blog

To the #lingeriechat ladies (you know who you are): you have been a veritable global font of information and support. I enjoy our tweetchat hours together.

Kudos and appreciation to the entire MUSE team from the Wharton School of Business, including marketing professor Keith Niedermeier, project goddess (although that might not be her official title) Brittany Shaw, Emily Sherbany, Sophia Coll, Dina Shteyngardt, and MUSE president Andrew Harrington. Your research and insights have been invaluable.

Finally, my deepest thanks to the friends who have let me ask every manner of personal questions about their bras. I couldn't have done this without you. You define the Fab in fabulous.

Ali Cudby
2011

About the Author

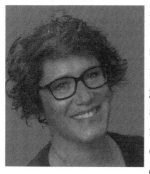 Ali Cudby's expertise as a bra coach began with her own journey. She spent her early bra-wearing years miserable when shopping in the lingerie department, as she was never able to find bras that fit. She was not alone – between 70% and 85% of women wear the wrong bras and can actually damage their health in the process. In 2004, Ali discovered a whole new world of bras and began developing her own fit technique.

As the CEO of Fab Foundations™ LLC, Ali's bra fit advice goes to tens of thousands of industry professionals each month. In addition to her writing, Ali works closely with manufacturers and retailers, studying buyer behavior, technological innovations in lingerie, and marketing opportunities.

Ali is a graduate of the University of Pennsylvania and the Wharton School of Business. Prior to founding Fab Foundations™, Ali owned an award-winning home building company. She has also held strategic marketing roles for The New York Times Company and the Animal Planet Television Network.

Ali lives in the Washington DC area with her husband, two teenagers and two dogs.

You can find Ali on Facebook at her Ali Cudby Author page and on Twitter @alicudby.

For more information on
Ali Cudby,
FabFoundations™
and Busted!
please visit
www.fabfoundations.com.

For media queries and orders,
please contact Fab Foundations™
at info@fabfoundations.com

Made in the USA
Charleston, SC
23 April 2013